Donation to the Post Graduate Center
in recognition of their contributions to make
this clinical account possible

DISORDERS OF THE LOWER GENITO URINARY TRACT SERIES

DISORDERS OF THE LOWER GENITO URINARY TRACT SERIES

SERIES EDITOR: A. R. MARKOS

Sexually Transmitted Diseases

A.R. Markos

2009. ISBN: 978-1-60741-584-8

DISORDERS OF THE LOWER GENITO URINARY TRACT SERIES

SEXUALLY TRANSMITTED DISEASES

A. R. MARKOS

Nova Biomedical Books

New York

Library of Congress Cataloging-in-Publication Data

Markos, A.R.
Sexually transmitted diseases / A.R. Markos.   p. cm.
Includes index.
ISBN 978-1-60741-584-8 (hardcover)
1. Sexually transmitted diseases. I. Title.
RC200.1.M37 2009, 616.95'1--dc22   2009013527

Published by Nova Science Publishers, Inc. ✦ *New York*

Contents

Preface

Disorders of the Lower Genito-Urinary Tract book series is intended to address the clinical and practical issues for conditions affecting female and male genital tract. The series will address Sexually Transmitted Diseases, Genital Dermatology and Sexual Dysfunctions under separate titles.

The emphasis will be on clinical skills and practical expertise; withdrawing from a cumulative thirty years experience in General Practice, Urology, Obstetrics & Gynaecology, Genital dermatology, Venereology and Sexual Dysfunction.

The current title will concentrate on Sexually Transmitted Infections (STIs). The book is not intended to be exhaustive or inclusive lists, but rather an overview of clinical and practical issues, relevant to the diagnosis and management of STIs, in primary and secondary care settings.

The recommendations I have laid in this book are intended to bring clinical and practical issues to the attention of the reader. They may not be appropriate for all clinical situations. The individual patient circumstances, the local resources and clinical judgement will influence the attending clinician's final decision of how to follow recommendations.

I have taken care to ensure that the listed drugs, dosages and routes of medication are correct. The prescribing physicians have duty to ensure the accuracy of the medication they prescribe and comply with their own licensing, regulatory and stautory rules. Clinical, investigative and therapeutic procedures require training, supervision and experience. The practicing clinican must learn from the learned experience of others; but critically appraise the methods of his own choice.

Introduction

The Prevalence of Sexually Transmitted Infections

The World Health Organisation (WHO) estimates that a million people acquire a sexually transmitted infection (STI), including the human immuno-deficiency virus (HIV), every day; the majority of whom are in low-income areas. The conditions affect all ages and social groups, with worse implications for the younger and poorer, due to lack of resources and/or access to diagnosis and treatment. The list includes more than 30 different organisms that are transmissible through intimate sexual contact (bacteria, viruses and/or parasites).The prevalence of individual conditions will be listed with the relevant disease.

There is a gap between industrialised and poor countries in available healthcare resources for the diagnosis, and/or treatment for STIs.this gap is wide and increasing. The levels of STI surveillance and control systems are variable, which suggests under-diagnosis and suboptimal management. There is also a gap in STI clinical care between different groups of people, in a given society. The young, socially deprived, females, ethnic minorities, mentally/physically handicapped, socially unstable, and/or patients with personality disorders are more vulnerable to STIs. The access of the socially disadvantaged and at risk groups to healthcare is low, if any at all; which leads to delayed diagnosis and treatment. It provides opportunity for complications, in the infected person, and spread to other contacts, by sexual transmission. The escalating coast of advanced technology makes the mere testing and objective microbiological /serological diagnosis of STIs under-resourced. This promotes the idea of treatment on clinical suspesions, without the objective support of investigations (e.g., Syndromic treatment). Treatment without objective and confirmed diagnosis carries the potential of erroneous diagnosis and the under-estimate of the real burden of the STI case load and complications, in the given community.

The Health Care and Social Cost of STIs

The burden of STIs reflects on interpersonal relationships, physical and mental health, industrial and agricultural productivity, economic standards and most important of all, human reproduction. There is a financial cost of treatable STIs, but the socio-economic burden of untreated STIs is incalculable. It is estimated that 19 million new STIs occur each year in the USA, almost half of them among 15-24 years old. The direct medical cost was estimated, in 2006, to be $14.7 billion annually. STIs and their consequences are one of the top five disease categories for which adults seek healthcare.

STIs are sinister because of the serious delayed consequences. STIs can lead to preventable serious complications like pelvic inflammatory disease, infertility, ectopic pregnancy and genital cancers (most notably cervical cancer in women). A third of female infertility is the consequence of post-inflammatory tubal damage. Women who suffer PID are 10 times more likely to develop ectopic pregnancy. Half of ectopic pregnancies can be attributed to previous PID. Pregnant women with untreated early syphilis would suffer 1 in 4 chances of stillbirth and 1 in 8 of neonatal death. The incidence is particularly relevant in areas of high prevalence of syphilis in pregnant women, like Africa, where up to 1 in 7 is infected. Serious ophthalmia naonatorum can affect 1 in 3 infants, newborn to mothers, with untreated Chlamydia or gonorrhoeal infection. STI could cause death, directly and indirectly, for the foetus, infants and adults. Tertiary Syphilis, chronic liver disease and liver failure are examples of the long term morbidities.

The impact of HIV on morbidity and mortality is significant across the globe. HIV is the commonest cause of young/adult death in Africa. The impact on the community is significant. There are 14 millions orphans due to AIDS; children and elders are left to care for each other. To date, it is estimated that 22million individuals died with AIDS and 42 millions are living with HIV/AIDS, most of whom are in sub-saharan Africa, and 19 millions are women. The associated immuno-suppression and opportunistic infections reduce productivity of young men, for months or years, and lead to premature death. In some areas one of three individuals is affected with HIV/AIDS.

The Influence of Globalisation and Travel on STIs

The ease of travel lead to the transfer of STI conditions from one geographical area to another. It can lead to the appearance of unusual STIs (e.g., a tropically acquired genital STI in patient/s living in an non-tropical areas). The clinician needs to map the prevalence of different STIs in the world in relation to the attending patient's risk factors.

The use of antibiotics is liberal in some communities, with availability of drugs over-the-counter and in non medical outlets. The problem of counterfeit drugs and/or preparations with substandard dosages should not be under-estimated. The improper or substandard use of antibiotics contributes to microbial resistance and requires clinical attention.Travellers to areas where STI drug resistance is a problem can bring the same infection to their homeland. Socioeconomic upheavals, associated with wars and mass immigration leads to social instability and break in interpersonal relations; which caries risks of commercial sex, casual and /or multiple sexual encounters.

The Clinical Provisions for the Management of STIs

The healthcare provisions for the diagnosis and treatment of STIs are variable in different parts of the world and often within the countries' healthcare economies. There are specialised clinics for the management of STIs in some countries. In the UK, The Venereal Diseases (VD) Clinics existed since 1920s. These evolved into Genito Urinary Medicine & Sexual Health Clinics, to improve public perception and reduce the stigma associated with VDs. In some European countries, Public Health Units provide diagnosis, treatment and contact tracing for STIs. Many other modalities of care are provided by different countries for the management of STIs; through specialists in Dermato-Venereology (Europe), physicians with special interests in venereology (USA), general practitioners and/or family doctors (Netherlands). The extent of contact tracing is also variable.

The management of STIs in UK benefits from dedicated clinics that provide free, confidential investigations.and treatment of STIs. The clinics have trained Health Advisors for patients support, counselling, contact tracing and partner notification. The clinics keep separate medical notes and patients' personal information. The clinics handle patients' investigations through separate identifying numbers, not names. The strict confidentiality fosters patients trust and help to bring individuals for STI tests, diagnoses and treatment; who may be otherwise reluctant to attend. The clinics code patients' diagnosis and STI and forward the records, on quarterly bases, to the Health Protection Agency, for public health records'. The understanding of epidemiological trends is advantageous in studying patterns of spread of STIs within communities, age groups, genders, sexual orientation, ethnicity and / or socio-economic sectors of society. This could better inform the targeting of health care resources and implementation of prevention and health education programes. The GUM clinics' staff network and communicate with each other, in confidentiality, to contact trace partner/s of an index case, even if s/he lived in another catchment area.

There is no perfect model of service that would suite every situation, country or group of individuals. The local professionals need to model and develop their own service according to the need of their client base and local circumstances.

The Common Organisms Causing Sexually Transmitted infections

Viruses:

- Human Immunodeficiency Virus (HIV)
- Herpes Simplex Virus (HSV1 & HSV2)
- Human Papilloma Virus (HPV)
- Molluscum Contagiosum Virus (MCV)
- Hepatitis A, B, C and D Viruses (Hep A, Hep B, Hep C & Hep D)
- Cytomegalovirus (CMV)
- Human Herpes Virus-8 (HHV8)

Bacteria:

- Neisseria gonorrhoeae
- Chlamydia trachomatis
- Treponema pallidum
- Haemophilus ducreyi
- Klebsiella (Calymmatobacterium) granulomatis

Parasites:

- Phthirus pubis
- Sarcoptes scabiei

Protozoa:

- Trichomonas vaginalis
- Amoeba & Giardia species

Fungi:

- Candida species (most commonly albicans)

Venereal Diseases are exclusively transmitted by sexual intercourse (e.g., Syphilis); others are transmitted by close and intimate contacts (e.g., parasitic infections).

The Principles of Managing Patients with STIs

1) The Patient

Individuals could be affected, directly or indirectly, by STIs. The innocent newborn may be affected by vertical transmission, from an infected mother and the unsuspecting person with infidelity of his/her cohabiting partner. Some conditions have extended periods of dormancy; with the clinical lesion appearing months or years after the original infection (e.g., syphilis, viral STIs).The physician has a role and responsibility in identifying patients who are at risk of STIs, for the proactive advice and offer of tests; as part of the clinical care and professional responsibility. There are clinical conditions that require consideration, as part of differential diagnosis and/or a proactive exclusion. For examples, there is a need to consider Chlamydial and/or Gonorrhoeal infections in the differential diagnosis of a patients with Pelvic Inflammatory Disease. Syphilis should be excluded in a young person presenting with cerebro-vascular accident, aortic aneurysm, personality changes and or neurological conditions. The clinician need to take action for proactive contact tracing of the sex partner/s of a patient with an infectious condition of serious consequences (e.g., HIV, Syphilis, Gonorrhoea); therefore contact/s of the index patient become potential STIs patients.

The clinician who cares for patients with STIs would have to deal with practical issues in challenging situations. The index patient may have had past exposure to STIs then received antibiotics, for another medical condition, leading to the incidental treatment ofhis/her STI. The sex partner may then get STI diagnosis but have no history of sexual risk activity. It will be a challenge to introduce the diagnosis of STIs to a patient who is not suspecting STIs. The unexpected diagnosis of STIs, in the non suspecting person, is usually met with disbelief and at times anger; which may be channeled at the medical staff. The clinician should encourage partners to communicate with each other. S/he should not divulge personal information reagarding one partner to the other; but maintain individual patients' confidentiality. Partners may chose to attend the consultation together; and the clinician should establish they understand the significance of their combined attendance and obtain their informed consent. The clinician should be non- judgemental and deal with the patients' problems sympathetically and empathetically. Clinical management of STIs require specialized clinician skills and sensitivities for handling the emotional and personal implications. The clinician should maintain scientific and professional honesty (i.e identifying the condition as sexuallty transmitted); whilest avoiding damage in relationship between the partners.

2) Clinical Assessment

Sexual history taking requires special expertise. The atmosphere of the consultation should be relaxed, confidential and non-judgemental. Clinical assessment proformas insures consistency and reflects formality. There will be patients who would feel embarrassed with elements of the sexual history and others who may volunteer details that are not necessary for clinical purposes. The skilful clinician should be able to bring either patient in line with sexual history necessary for clinical care. The patient should be given the opportunity to express her/his own request/complaint in his own words. Many patients request "a check". The subsequent enquiry about "the reason of concern" opens an opportunity for the patient and the clinician for a detailed sexual history.

The general clinical skills of keeping eye contact, listening carefully and observing non-verbal cues should be applied. Sexual health patients are usually apprehensive and perceptive. Some bring another person for assurance. The clinician should make the patient aware of issues of confidentiality and be conscious of how the presence of a third party might limit the patient's divulgence of information. The clinician should not use leading questions and avoid medical jargon.

Basic information includes the last sexual contact, any other sex contacts within the previous year, sexual practice (ie. Vaginal, genito-oral, oro-genital and/or rectal sex) and sexual orientation. The patient needs to understand that the sexual practice dictates the orifices from which microbiological samples/swabs are required. Patient's incorrect denial of a sexual practice could circumvent tests that are necessary for making the correct diagnosis. For example, rectal examination is not indicated in a patient who denies rectal sex or has no corresponding symptoms. Rectal conditions could otherwise be missed, if the patient inaccurately denies the practice of receptive rectal sex.

The examination room should be confidential and comfortable, for both patients and staff. A seprate patient changing room/ toilet maintains client's own privacy. It is wise to have a chaperone, irrespective of the sex of the patient and that of the attending clinician. Clinicians requires an opportunity to speak to the patient on his/her own, to obtain any additional information, that otherwise could had been restricted by the presence of a third party (e.g., sex partner). It is essential to obtain an informed consent, for each examination and/or test. The clinician should not assume consent. The mere presence of the patient in the sexual health clinic does not imply that he/she is giving consent for genital, pelvic, rectal examination and/or tests. It is important to promote the patients confidence and co-operation by explanation. Pressure may lead a patient to take a test but decline the follow up advice. Eventually, any test result will be of value if the patient co-operates with the clinical advice advice.

Inspection should be through, to identify genital discharge, skin changes, lesions and/or parasites. A good light is essential and the help of a magnifying lens may be necessary. The patient can pinpoint the area of concern and this can also show how s/he is comfortable or otherwise with the genitalia. All skin folds must be inspected thoroughly. The male patients' retraction of his own prepuce avoids unnecessary pain. The lithotomy position allows for the inspection of the perianal area in females. Vaginal speculum examination gives an opportunity to inspect the vaginal wall and cervix; and is essential for vaginal and cervical samples, without which the assessment is not complete. Proctoscopy and inspection of the lower rectum and anal area is indicated in patients who have rectal symptoms or admitted to rectal intercourse; hence the necessity of accurate history. The presence of discharge can direct to a provisional diagnosis and should direct the investigations. Mucopurulent discharge is suggestive of gonorrhoeal infection but severe Chlamydial disease can lead to copious discharge simulating mucopurulent one. The typical discharge of vaginal Candidiasis or Trichomoniasis can lend itself to provisional diagnosis and should be supported by laboratory investigations, which also confirm or exclude concurrent infections. Lesions should be described and recorded (i.e site, size, shape, colour, consistency…). A sketch drawing of lesions facilitates the follow-up care.Inspection of other body parts may be necessary in some cases (e.g., mouth and throat in patient with history of oral sex, symptoms and/or lesions)

Palpation of the inguinal area is done as routine. The finding of inguinal lymph nodes is not uncommon, as they drain the lower limbs in addition to external genitalia. Their presence is significant in acute herpetic attacks, syphilis and lympho- granuloma. Scrotal examination is important as the majority of patients are young and within the age of testicular tumours. Any suspicious lesion should proceed to testicular ultrasonography. Epididymal cysts are usually innocent and the patient should be assured. Epididymal/testicular tenderness is significant for cases of Epididymo-orchitis. Bi-manual pelvic examination in females is essential part of the assessment for pelvic pain and/or dyspareunia. The clinical findings could support or exclude the possibility of pelvic inflammatory disease. The finding of pelvic mass should proceed to request ultra-sonography. Ovarian cysts in the young are usually innocent and regress on follow up ultra-sonography. Ovarian lesions in middle and senior age should be seriously considered; due to the insidious nature of incidental ovarian cancer.

3) At site basic laboratory procedures

Gram-staining, microscopy testing and urinalysis help to support the diagnosis of male Urethritis, female Cervicitis, Candidiasis, Trichomoniasis and Bacterial vaginosis. Some 50% of Gonorrhoea in female cervicitis/urethritis and 90% in male urethritis could be diagnosed with Gram-staining and microscopy. The same day provisional diagnosis, treatment and sexual helth advice to abstain from sexual intercourse and contact tracing are practical benefits that both patients and clinicians appreciate.

The *male urethral swab* is better obtained by a plastic loop, which could be moistened with sterile water, to facilitate insertion and collection of sample. Cotton tipped swabs are used by some clinics. The swab should be inserted to at least 3 cm in depth, to bypass the distal part of the urethra, which is lined by stratified epithelium. The urethral sample is then smeared on a glass slide, for Gram-staining and microscopy. The identification of "Gram- Negative Intracellular Diplococci" (GNID) helps the provisional diagnosis and initiation of treatment in some 90% of positive cases of Gonorrhoeal urethritis. The same loop/sample is used for a spread on a microbiology culture plate for the purpose of N gonorrhoeae culture and susceptibility to antibiotics. A secondary urethral swab used to be the norm for Chlamydia test samples, when Enzyme Immuno Assay (EIA) tests were in use. The current Nucleic Acid Amplification Test (NAAT), is validated for Chlamydia testing in male urine samples. Micturition, before the urethral swab, may remove the discharge and lead to a false negative test. Clinicians should advice patients to avoid urination, for two hours before the urethral tests

Urinalysis help to identify cases of urethritis, cystitis and other urinary tract infections (UTIs). The dip-stick test is widely available; but urine centrifuge and microscopy could also provide valuable results. The first catch urine sample, if positive for polymorph-nuclear White Blood Cells (WBCs) and/or Nitrates, help the diagnosis of urethritis. If the second catch urine sample is positive; a mid stream one should be sent for microbiology microscopy, culture and sensitivity tests. If there is evidence of haematuria, gross or microscopic, then renal tract ultrasonography and urethra-cystoscopy are indicated, to exclude underlying lesions. A false reading of haematuria may follow the urethral swband in severe inflammation; and should be verified at another opportunity. It is not uncommon to diagnose Diabetes Mellitus first following the identification of glycosuria in association with Balano-posthitis. Significant proteinuria should alert the clinician to the possibility of rare but clinically serious glomerulo-nephritis. UTIs are common in females; but should lead investigations to exclude underlying pathology in the renal tract in a male patient. Renal tract ultra-sonography, should be ordered as the first step; and may be followed by cysto-urethro-scopy, according to the patient's age.

Vaginal swabs and slide samples for Gram- staining and microscopy, help the diagnosis of Candidiasis and support that of Cervicitis (ie in the presence of leucorrhoeae/WBCs). A second vaginal sample, mixed on a glass slide with normal saline, is obtained for microscopic assessment and can help the diagnosis of Trichomoniasis. Samples from the cervical canal, for Gram- staining and microscopy, can give early identification of "Gram- Negative Intracellular Diplococci" (GNID) in some 50% of positive cases of Gonorrhoeal cervicitis. The cervical swab is also spread on a microbiological plate for N gonorrhoeae culture and antibiotic susceptibility. EIA tests for Chlamydia required intra-cervical material to obtain columnar epithelial cells, which harbour the organism. Visualisation of the cervix and external os were, therefore, necessary. The availability and sensitivity of NAAT for Chlamydia has made it easier to obtain samples (e.g high vaginal and self samples). NAAT are also available for N gonorrhoeae, but antibiotic susceptibility tests continue to be required. There is little clinical value in the wide-spread and routine use of "High Vagilal Swabs", for non specific microbiology culture tests.

Microscopy examination, of cells scraped from genital ulcer suspected for Herpes Genitalis, could support the diagnosis; on the finding of multi-nucleate giant cells; which may also be found when cervical cytology encounter an incidental lesion. The availability of Polymerase Chain Reaction (PCR) for Herpes Virus is leading to earlier and accurate diagnosis; which is clinically valuable.

Dark Ground Microscopy is useful for the early diagnoses, and consequently early treatment and contact tracing, of syphilis. On site testing for Chlamydia and HIV are under-way; but quality controls are a concern. A false positive or false negative test would have high medical and social consequences. The tests are time consuming but worth-while in remote areas, where patients return for treatment and follow up is an issue.

4) Screening for STIs

The concept of screening lends itself well to the control of STIs. The conditions are widespread, prevalent, have serious public health consequences, have reliable tests and cost effective therapeutics. Screening pregnant women for HIV, Syphilis and Hepatitis B is part of the national ante-natal screening care in the UK. A new programme for screening young women for Chlamydia, in UK, is underway, with increasing demand to make it annual practice and extend it to young men. There are also sporadic programmes for offering HIV, Syphilis, Hep B and Hep C screening to men having sex with men (MSM), in gay saunas, nightclubs and outreach services for sex workers. Screening for STIs, in at risk population is useful in identifying those who are at risk but unsuspecting, and otherwise may not request STI investigations.

5) Testing for STIs

The improved sex education in western societies coupled with libral attitudes and multiplicity of sexual partners, initiate patients to request "sexual health check to exclude STIs". The patient expectation sets the boundries of professional and medico-legal responsibility, on the attending clinician, to offer:

1. Assessment and investigations for all STIs, and
2. Tests within the condition's own incubation and/or window periods.
3. Proactive management of diagnosed and/or potential STIs, for the index patient and sex partner/s

Patients, who present with a condition that is sexually transmitted, need assessment and tests, to exclude other STIs. One-third of patients diagnosed with STI, on average, would have another concurrent condition of sexually related significance. As a principle, when there is patient concern of one STI, s/he should be offered test and exclude other STIs. *The tests should aim to make the diagnosis and/or exclusion of all STIs.*

A patient who attends within few hours of sexual contact and exposure to STIs, require tests according to the conditions, own incubation and window periods (ie after one and two weeks, for N.gonorrhoea and C. trachomatis and three months for HIV, Syphilis and Hepatitis B). Another patient who attends before the window periods for serology tests, would require repeat serum sample after the three months window period, calculated from the date of exposure.During this period, the patient's status could be a potential risk to other sex contacts, if s/he is harbouring undiagnosed condition.

6) Contact Tracing and Partner Notification

STIs are communicable diseases, acquired by intimate sexual contact. It is a public health responsibility to seek to identify the sexual contact for advice, investigations and treatment. The aim is to treat those affected and break the cycle of further contagious spread. This could start with encouraging the incumbent patient of contacting the sex partner/s (*Index Patient Contact Tracing*). In UK, the GUM clinic provide a *"Contact Slip"* which records the index patient's clinic identity number, not name or date of birth; the STIs diagnostic code and the clinic's name. The index patient is advised to forward the Contact Slip/s to the sex partner/s; to take to the nearest GUM clinic. Contact Slips allow the cross matching of partners' details and infections and help a distant clinic to identify the STIs affecting the index case; and therefore the care required for the contact. The success or otherwise of this process is variable with the socio-cultural backgrounds and individual couples' situation. It is not possible to speculate who acquired the STIs first in a relationship; and, on many occasions, the length of time that lapsed from infection to diagnosis. The frequent use of antibiotics means that some STIs may be incidentally treated. It is possible that a patient acquired an infection first, transmited it to his/her partner, received antibiotic therapy for another medical condition; which incidentally treats the STI, leaving the unsuspecting partner with a positive diagnosis and no other explanation. Viral STIs may also have a protracted period of dormancy and sub-clinical presentations. Genital Herpes is becoming more common of HSV Type I, and could be acquired between two partners in a steady relationship, through oral sex.

In similar scenarios, it would be incorrect and professionally improper to imply or withdraw a conclusion of infidelity,of the diagnosed patient.

The index patient may have lost communication with the sex contact; which makes contact tracing impossible. There is a public health duty, to control contagious infections and avoid or curtail their spread. In the absence of a communication channel (e.g., partner's name, address and/ or telephone number), the health advisors are not able to fulfil contact tracing. If the health advisor/visitor can establish channels of communication, they will be able to contact trace the partner/s *(Provider Based Contact Tracing)*. The process is time and resource intensive. It should be used as a secondary line, if and when index patient based contact tracing fails (or declined by the index patient).

There are situations when the index patient continue to have intercourse with a known partner (e.g., wife/ husband), exposing her/him to a serious infection. It could be argued that the incumbent health care professionals have a duty of care to warn the unsuspecting partner. This issue is legally complicated and the health carers need clarifications from their own professional bodies.

7) Medico Legal Issues

There had been patients who discovered that STIs were the cause of their symptoms, became furiously angry and looked for redress with the sex partner. There had been legal suits, in Western societies, when the infected person brought legal proceedings against the sex partner, for causing "Grievous Bodily Harm". There were also legal suits brought by affected patient, against healthcare professionals, for "failing to properly advice on the possibility and/or modality of transmission of STIs". The clinician need to offer clear advice to patients with STIs, regarding the modes of transmission and possibility of causing infection and/or harm to sex partner/s.

8) Sexual Assault, Rape, Child Sexual Abuse and STIs

Rape and/or sexual assault is a legal judgement and for judge and jury to decide. The clinician's main duty is to provide clinical care for the patient/victim. The definition of rape is legally guided and may vary from one country to another (e.g., many countries now define the non-consensual penetration of the mouth by a penis or vagina by a finger as rape). Some reports suggest that 1 in 4 women have experienced rape or attempted rape; the vast majority of whom (up to 90%) have not reported the incident. Of those who report the assault to the police, a small proportion (5-10%), have the assailant convicted. These data relate to western industrialised countries.There are no or little information from developing societies. Men who experience sexual assault and/or buggery are less likely to report the incident to the police. The medical attendant my be called to court, as *witness of fact*, to testify on medical findings. S/he should balance her/his duty of care, sympathy and empathy to the patient in distress, with impartiality, neutrality, accuracy and objectivity.

The transmission of STIs is a concern for victims of sexual assault, rape and/or child sexual abuse. The clinician's duty is to the patient/victim, for the diagnosis, exclusion and treatment of STIs. The treatment may be therapeutic and/or prophylactic. The clinician has a medico-legal duty to undertake samples with forensic interests in mind. It is in the patient's own interest that the examination and test samples are conducted by a professional who is familiar with forensic procedures, and should follow a strict guidelines and protocols. In the UK, this is usually conducted in *specialised sexual assault/rape units* or by a "police surgeon". Most patients request the assessment by a female staff (e.g police officer, doctor, nurse, health advisor and/or psychologist). The patient wishes must be respected.

The attending physician needs to provide an atmosphere of understanding, sympathy and empathy. The recording of signs should be meticulous, impartial and unbiased. Recording with diagrams, photographs and magnification (e.g., colposcopy) is valuable for objective recording.

The clinician need to handle first the psychological and/or physical trauma, before attending to the question of STIs. Some STIs are not amenable to diagnosis, except after a significant period of time (e.g., serology tests for HIV, Syphilis and/or Hep B will require a window period of three months). The incubation period of STIs influences the timing and validity of the tests (e.g., it may be necessary to repeat culture tests for N gonorrhoea after 1, 2 and 3 weeks). HIV Post Exposure Prophylaxis should be considered within the first 48 hours after the incident, possibly longer. There is a place for antibiotic therapy/prophylaxis, against Gonorrhoea, Chlamydia and Syphilis and an accelerated course of Hepatitis B vaccination. There are benefits with the Human Gama-Globulins (HGG); but their availability is restricted.

9) Clinical Practicalities for managing sexual assault

1. Forensic samples and tests are required before any attempted clinical assessment; which may interfere with the validity of the samples (e.g., a vaginal swab may remove an important forensic material of sperms and/or DNA).

2. The clinician should proactively enquire whether the patient have reported the case to the police, or intending to do so, to give the police surgeon the first opportunity to obtain forensic samples.

3. The explicit timing and orifice/s assaulted is important for the selection of type and site of swaps (e.g rectal swap are necessary following buggery). The clinician should identify the possible route of transmission of infection/s; consequently the site and type of test samples.

4. Emotional and psychological support is important throughout the process of history taking and examination. The experience of specialised and dedicated staff is valuable.

5. The clinician's sympathetic and empathetic role, in interacting with the patient's condition, should be balanced with an accurate and precise record of findings. Over-emphasising observations could prove counterproductive in a court of law, if there is evidence of bias.

6. Neither the presence of STIs or injuries is required legally to judge a case of rape. Rape and sexual assault may take place without any evidence of injuries, including genital signs. Injuries may take place during consensual intercourse and, therefore, on their own are not evidence of rape. A victim of rape may have a pre-existing STI and an assailant may be free of STIs.

7. The identification of STIs in a child should raise the question of Child Sexual Abuse (CSA). The area is complex and better dealt with by a specialised team. A *Child Protection Team* would benefit from the expertise of a specialised Paediatrician, Family Doctor, Paediatric Nurse, Social Worker and STD clinician.

8. Every sample handler should sign, date and record the time of the sample, with the subsequent handler, clinicians and microbiologists included. All staff should keep a *"chain of evidence"*.

9. The clinician may be called by court as a *"witness of fact"*; to report her/his observations and findings.

10. The court may request the expertise of an independent doctor or scientist, to act as *"Expert Witness"*; whose exclusive duty is to court not to either parties of claimant or defendant
11. The clinician should keep a clear, contemporaneous comprehensive and legible account of findings.
12. Culture for N gonorrhoea and C trachomatis are required for medico-legal purposes. NAAT tests are helpful for clinical management, but have not been scrutinized for court purposes.

The Human Papilloma Virus (HPV) Infections and Genital Warts

Prevalence

Genital Human Papilloma Virus (HPV) infection is the most common STI. The American Center for Disease Control and Prevention (CDC) estimates that 50% of sexually active men and women acquire genital HPV infection at some time and over 6 million new infections each year. The reports of the UK Health Protection Agency (HPA), indicates that in 2006, 83,745 new cases of genital warts were diagnosed; with rates ranging between 150-200/100,000 population, varying with sex and county of residence. Up to 1 in 4 of young adults has evidence of the HPV virus. The majority of patients (up to 90%) infected with HPV do not develop clinical lesions (i.e., warts). Sub-clinical lesions are common but not necessary to identify, as it would be impractical to aim for the eradication of Sub-clinical lesions. Eventually, the patient's own immune system combats the HPV infection, in 90% of the cases, within two years.

The Virus

HPV is an icosahedral envelop (*capsid*), containing double stranded DNA structure. The viron is 55 nm in diameter, and lends itself to detection by Polymerase Chain Reaction (PCR); which is used for identification and typing. There are more than 100 HPV types, 40 of which infect the skin and/or mucus membranes of the vulva, vagina, cervix, anus, penis and/or rectum. HPV types have predilection to specific sites. Some HPV types have a potential to induce cancer (*Oncogenic HPV*) and are considered of "high risk" (e.g., HPV 16, 18), as compared with other types that cause genital warts and considered of "low risk" (e.g., HPV 6, 11).

Transmission

Close genital skin to skin contacts, including genital fluids, is the main method of transmission. It is aided by minor skin abrasions. It does not require penetrative sex and may take place in an area that is not covered by a condom. Transmission can take place from hand warts into the genital area (*Auto-inoculation*); but is rare. This is hypothesised by the observation of HPV types that have a predilection to general skin, causing warts in the genital area and vice-versa. Oro-genital transmission is recognised. The infection could also be passed from mother to baby, during vaginal delivery (*Vertical transmission*).

Presentation and Diagnosis

The majority of patients present with cosmetic concerns, regarding the appearance of the warty lesion/s. The finding of a foreign genital growth can alarm the patient and/or partner. The patients' emotional reactions are exaggerated by the knowledge of the sexual nature of transmission and correlation to genital cancers. The clinician should target clinical care to minimise anxiety, provide assurance in addition to lesional management.

The lesions could be single or multiple, flat or cauliflower in shape, coloured with the skin or pigmented. Some lesions are associated with soreness (e.g., inguinal, perineal and peri-anal warts) others with bleeding (urethral, anal, vaginal and/or cervical). The diagnosis is clinical in most of the cases and the majority of lesions. The application of cotton / gauze soaked with 5% acetic acid, to a lesion suspicious of wart (*Acetic Acid Test*), lead to the reversible conversion of the lesion to a whitish colouration (*Aceto-white*). The test could be used as a non-specific bedside test. Flat lesions may simulate Intraepithelial Neoplasia and deserve a special attention; as the management and follow-up care are significantly different. Inspecting small lesions could be aided with magnification and better lighting (Colposcopy, Vulvoscopy, Penoscopy and Anoscopy). Biopsy is rarely necessary. Biopsy has a role in pigmented lesions, to exclude melanotic changes, and in flat lesions, to exclude Intra-epithelial Neoplasia. Giant warts are rare and should have the benefit of excision biopsy and histology; to identify the locally invasive *Buschke and Lowenstein Tumour*, which have a potential for malignant transformation. HPV typing has no clinical value for the management of genital warts. HPV typing has gained clinical value in identifying women at risk of Cervical Intra-epithelial Neoplasia (CIN). Patients harbouring oncogenic HPV types require closer and more frequent cytology/colposcopy observations.

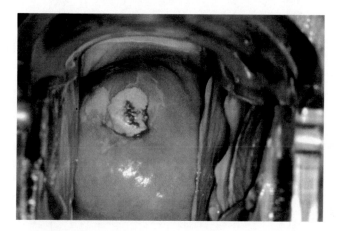

Figure 1. Cervical Wart

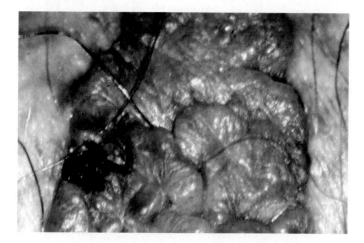

Figure 2. Compound Naevus

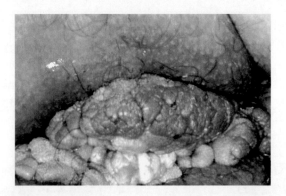

Figure 3. Giant Perianal Warts

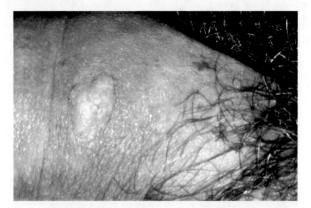

Figure 4. Penile Wart

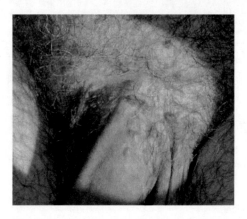

Figure 5. Penile Warts at area not covered with Condom

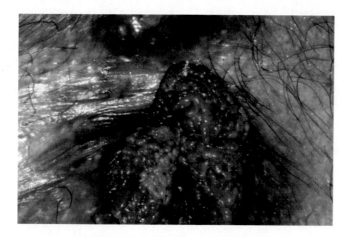

Figure 6. Large Perianal wart

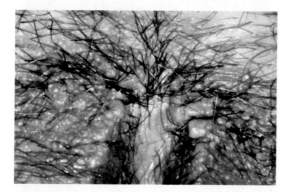

Figure 7. Multiple Perianal warts

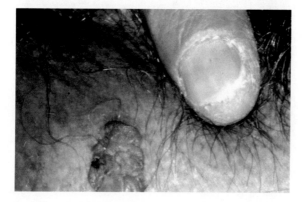

Figure 8. Pigmented wart

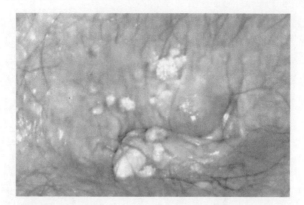

Figure 9. Small perianal warts

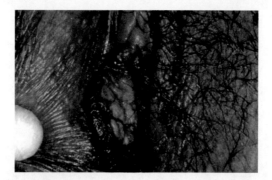

Figure 10. Vulval Intra- Epithelial Neoplasia (VIN)

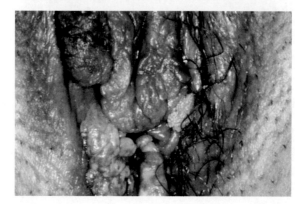

Figure 11. Vulval Warts

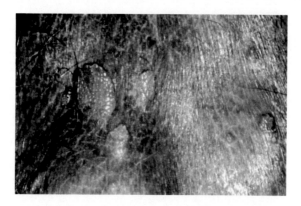

Figure 12. Vulval Warts associated with Vulval Intra- Epithelial Neoplasia (VIN)

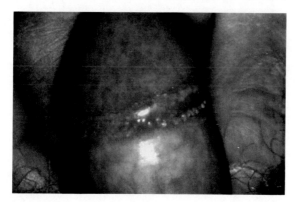

Figure 13. Pearly Penile papules

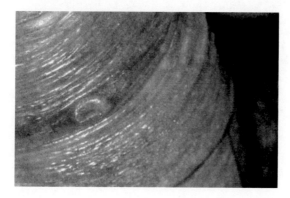

Figure 14. Penile papules

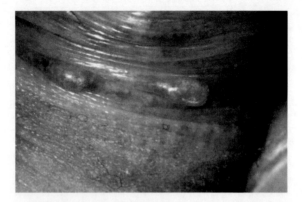

Figure 15. Penile papules

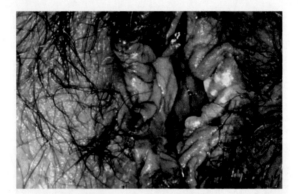

Figure 16. Vulval Intra- Epithelial Neoplasia (VIN) associated with warts

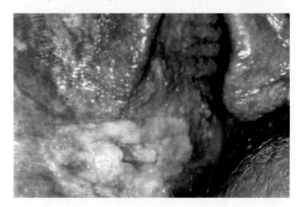

Figure 17. Vulval Intra- Epithelial Neoplasia (VIN): flat lesion

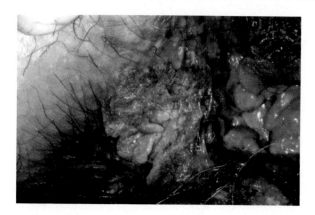

Figure 18. Vulval Intra- Epithelial Neoplasia (VIN): warty lesion

Differential Diagnosis

The clinical appearance of warts is diagnostic in most of the lesions. Innocent skin changes could be confused with genital warts for the inexperienced eye: Pearly Penile Papules, Vulval Papillae, genital Sebaceous Glands, prominent Hair Follicles, Skin Papillae/Tags and Cervical Nabothian Follicles are examples of innocent lesions that could be confused with warts.

The diagnosis of a genital lesion as wart is fulfilled only when the differential diagnosis of Intraepithelial Neoplasia, and consequently squamous cell and basal cell carcinoma, is completed. The increasing incidence of Syphilis requires attention, to exclude Condylomata Lata. These conditions should be proactively considered and excluded; for their serious consequences. Other less serious but clinically important conditions that require differential diagnosis include: Seborrhoeic Keratosis, Molluscum Contagiosum, Dermatofibroma, Angiokeratoma and Lichen Planus.

Practical Issues

1. The incubation period for genital warts could be protracted and lead to the surprise discovery of lesions in a patient who has had no suspicious sexual history for years, prior to the symptoms (eg. appearance of warts in the elderly or during pregnancy). This may raise issues regarding infidelity, and subsequent suspicions between the partners. The changing

immunological status of pregnancy or advancing age lead to the activation of a dormant or sub-clinical lesion and appearance of warts.
2. Flat lesions should be considered for biopsy; to exclude Intraepithelial Neoplasia, which is rarer than genital warts but require a different course of management.

Treatment

The main purpose of treatment for genital warts is cosmetic. The commonality of sub-clinical lesions (e.g., 5-10 lesions for every clinically identifiable wart), indicates that there will continue to be a reservoir of HPV, with the possibility of shedding. Aiming for the eradication of genital HPV and sub-clinical lesions is impractical. Different modalities of treatment aim to destroy the wart tissue by method of cyto- toxicity (Podophyllotoxin), chemical ablation (Trichloracetic acid), thermal ablation (Cryo-cautery or diathermy), tissue evaporation (LASER) and/or Immuno-modulator (Imiquimod 5%). All modalities have a potential for side-effects and associated with variable degrees of success or failure. The patient needs to be aware about the possibility of scarring and/or change in pigmentation at the site of treatment; to which young male patients are emotionally sensitive.

The choice of treatment should be the result of the patient/doctor interaction. The consideration of the lesion, its site, treatment options, their side-effects, complications and local resources, direct the patient/doctor decision algorithm. The patient's autonomy and choice should be respected, in balance with the available services and resources. Most patients would prefer home treatment (e.g., Podophyllotoxin or Imiquimod). Some patients prefer one-off treatment (e.g., diathermy, hyfrecation or laser); rather than the repeated episodes of clinic visits (e.g., Cryotherapy). Excision remains an option for solitary, large and long-standing warts. Excision is indicated for giant lesions suggestive of Buschke and Lowenstein tumour. An excision biopsy could be of diagnostic and therapeutic value for Intraepithelial Neoplasia.The different modalities have risks to users and patients; therefore training on their use and health and safety rules should be closely applied.

Most patients respond to treatment and very few remain with calcitrant lesions. Recurrences and new lesions may appear after treatment, irrespective of the modality. The patient should be warned that subclinical lesions may develop later into overt warts. The response to treatment is slow in smokers.

Modalities of Treatment

1. Topical Cytotoxics and necrotic agents:

Podophyllotoxin: The preparation has selective anti-mitotic and cytotoxicity activity, which leads to tissue necrosis. The preparation is available in solution form (0.5% in alcoholic basis), for painting lesions and cream (0.15%), which is suitable for areas not amenable for painting (e.g., vulval and peri-anal). It could be used at clinic and at home (i.e self application). The response rate is better with non-keratinized warts; due to ease of penetration of the active substance into the cells. The surrounding tissue is affected to variable degrees and rarely with aggressive hypersensitivity reactions, inflammation and ulceration. The patient should be aware of the possibilities of reactions and side effects. When there are complications, the patient should give particular attention to genital hygiene and topical antiseptic applications, to avoid secondary infection. The clinician should forewarn the patient on complications and their care. Podophyllotoxin should be avoided in pregnancy; and in women with unsafe contraception, who may become pregnant during the course of treatment.

Cryotherapy leads to vaso constriction, tissue hypoxia, cytolysis and inflammation. The choice of equipment depends on local supplies and range from disposable or reusable liquid nitrogen spray flasks, nitrous oxide or carbon dioxide cylinders and probes. The operator should aim to apply the probe or spray up to 2-3 seconds; which is usually guided by the patient's tolerance and acceptability. The patient's threshold for pain is a leading factor in treatment. The clinician may apply local anaesthetic cream (e.g., Emla Cream), topically to the wart area, some 15 min prior to the treatment episode.The cream lends itself to self application. If the local anaesthetic is medically introduced (e.g., sub-cutaneous infiltration with Lignocaine, 1or 2%), it opens the avenue of choice between Cryotherapy and other more ablative methods (e.g., Hyfrecation or Diathermy). It is remarkable how patients are prepared to tolerate genital pain associated with Cryotherapy, in their desire to get rid of warts.

Trichloracetic Acid (TCA) causes chemical coagulation followed by necrosis to the area of application. A very fine probe should be used to apply TCA, concentrations of 60-90%, on the warty changes and avoid the surrounding normal skin. It could be selectively used to destroy the keratinised coverings of warts, prior to the patient's attempts of home application of Podophyllotoxin or Imiquimod cream. The keratinised and dead tissue, could act as a barrier, hindering access of the active material to the viable wart tissue. TCA application removes the keratinized layer and achieves better access of Podophyllotoxin to the viable wart tissue.

Podophyllin Resin is a plant resin. Dissolved in alcohol (15-25%), it could be used for treatment, in cost conscious settings. Some of its components have teratogenic and oncogenic effects, which is a drawback to its use. The material was widely used, for decades, in GUM clinics, prior to the availability of Podophyllotoxin. There is no evidence of clinical cases with oncogenic changes. Neither the Podophyllin resin nor Podophyllotoxin should be considered during pregnancy, or in young women who have no safe contraception.

2. Electro therapy:tissue destruction by the electro-induced heat

- Hyfrecation (low power electricity)
- Electro-cautery (electrical heat application)
- Diathermy (high power electrical current that requires a diathermy pad)

3. Light Amplification of Stimulated Emission of Radiation (LASER)

LASER produces tissue destruction by evaporisation. It leaves less charring, than thermal methods; which aids quicker tissue recovery and healing.It provides an alternative for therapy, but no remarkable benefit over the advanced modalities of electro cautery and diathermy.

4. Topical immuno-modulator (Imiquimod 5% Cream)

The topical application stimulates the local immune-response and leads to topical inflammatory reactions, expressing itself in irritation, burning sensation and/or ulceration. The inflammatory response may be severe and complicate treatment, leading the patient to stop application. Patients find Imiquimod convenient, due to self application. Clinicians value its use for patients with reduced response to other methods.

5. Surgical excision

Surgical excision remains an option for solitary and large lesions. Some patients prefer a single episode of treatment, over recurrent clinic visits. Surgery may not feasible in multiple wide-spread lesions. It could be disappointing, to the patient and clinician, in case of recurrence of warts. The procedure is time, staff and resource intensive than home and self – treatment. It is necessary when there is suspension of Intra-epithelial Neoplasia and for large lesion suggestive of Buschke-Lowenstien Tumour.

Local Anaesthesia for Wart Treatment

The clinician must be perceptive to the patient's expression of pain and be led by the patient's response. Topical application of Emla Cream could be used successfully for local anaesthesia in most of the cases. Subcutaneous infiltration with Lignocaine (1or 2%) will be required for some patients. The prior application of anaesthetic cream (e.g., Emla) could ease the pain of subcutaneous infiltration. The depth and effectiveness of the anaesthetic could be assessed by testing the treatment site, by a needle prick or test application of the chosen method (e.g., cryotherapy), prior to the start of the procedure. Local anaesthesia is required prior to LASER, Hyfercation, Electro-cautery and diathermy; and may be needed before Cryo-therapy.

Recurrence of Genital Warts and Calcitrant Lesions

The majority of patients with early lesions will respond well to the different modalities of treatment. Clinical experience plays a part in selecting the right application for the right lesion and the agreeable patient. Longstanding lesions that have been neglected for protracted periods of time are usually calcitrant to treatment. Heavy smoking is associated resistance to treatment, leading to protracted course of lesions; and high recurrences following the initial respons to therapy. There is also individual patient factors; which need clinical management to menimise distress with lack of response or recurrences.

HPV Vaccine

The HPV vaccine is licensed for use in young females; to reduce the effect of Oncogenic HPV Types, and their risk in developing cervical cancer. There are two commercially available and licensed brands, a quadruple vaccine (type specific for HPV 6, 11, 16, 18), and a double vaccine (type specific for HPV16, 18). As a consequence of the vaccine, it is likely that the overall incidence and prevalence of genital warts may decline. The overall effect of the HPV vaccine on genital warts (i.e., reduction in incidence and prevalence), may be counteracted by a liberal sexual relationships, with consequent surge in HPV propagation. The final outcome could be a balancing effect, between an increasing prevalence of HPV infections, against any reduction caused by the HPV vaccination.

Clinical Practicalities

1. The appearance of genito-anal warts in a patient suggests sexual transmission. The doctor should offer assessment and investigation to exclude other STIs.

2. The sex partner would also benefit from assessment and investigations to exclude STIs.

3. The period between sexual contact, acquisition of HPV and the appearance of clinical lesion is variable. In clinical situations it is not possible to extrapolate from whom or when the lesion was acquired.

4. The relationship between HPV and cervical cancer is in the public domain. This can lead to anxiety, regarding the possibility of developing cancer. HPV lesions and genital warts are very common; whilst genital cancers and pre-cancerous conditions are less common. The clinician should be sensitive to the patient's concerns and address them with explanation The patient who undertakes regular cervical screening should not be unduly concerned. Cervical warts should be managed in parallel with regular and routine cervical cytology.

5. Genital warts alone are not indication for cervical cytology, but it would be unwise to use destructive methods for a cervical lesion, that is presumed to be a wart, without excluding underlying or concomitant Cervical Intraepithelial Neoplasia (CIN). Excision biopsy for cervical warts should be considered for therapeutic and diagnostic reasons.

6. Flat lesions may mimic Intra-epithelial Neoplasia; and excision biopsy has value in making a definitive diagnosis. A therapeutic test could be used for a defined short period (e.g., Podophyllotoxin topical application to the lesion first for few weeks). A non responsive lesion should then be submitted to biopsy to exclude Intra-epithelial Neoplasia.

7. Pregnancy could be associated with the appearance of a dormant or sub-clinical lesion or the exaggerations of an already existing growth. This can cause alarm to the woman and attending midwifes. Most patients request treatment during pregnancy. Cryotherapy is the method of choice; and is acceptable to most clinicians and patient. Drugs of teratogenic potential (eg. Podophyllotoxin) are contraindicated during pregnancy. Other topical applications are not licensed during pregnancy. The use of a treatment modality that requires anaesthesia during pregnancy is cumbersome.

8. Urethral/meatal warts tend to require more episodes of treatment than similar lesions in other sites. They also have a potential for recurrences. Different treatment modalities could be applied. The patient would need to increase his water intake, to encourage micturition, which opens the urethra meatus and prevent continuous contact of the urethral surfaces; to avoid adhesions. An antiseptic cream should be frequently used, by self application, to achieve separation of the opposing surfaces of the urethra.

9. The use of destructive methods to treat warts in one site, can accelerate the recovery and response to treatment in other sites. This is observable in the regression of anal, vaginal, and/or cervical warts, following the treatment of external genital lesions.The change of the antigenecity of the primary wart, caused by the destructive methods, enhances the patient's immune response to the altered new antigens, promoting the response in the other sites.

10. Opposing surfaces may coalesce and amalgamate with adhesions, if wart tissue destruction leads to opposing ulcerations (Kissing Ulcers). This should be observed for warts in the sub-preputial sac, urethral meatus and opposing vulval lips. The clinician should excersie a choice of treatment modality, elaborate explanation of post treatment care and choice of a patient who would adheres to medical advice. The patient needs instructions on the separation of the two surfaces, cleansing and the application of antiseptic cream, to avoid direct row surfaces contacts, adhesions and amalgamation.

Molluscum Contagiosum

Molluscum contagiosum (MC) is caused by a large DNA poxvirus, with two main sub-types MCV-I, with more predeliction to affect children, and MCV-II affecting more adults and HIV patients. Transmission occurs by skin-to-skin contact. Warm, humid environment and small skin abrasions encourages transmission and spread. Auto-inoculation can take place by scratching the lesion and transmission of the infected material, by finger nails, to another skin site. Generalised and widespread lesions are likely to affect children and patients with impaired immunity (e.g., HIV). Crops of multiple lesions should raise the suspicion of immuno-compromised status. Like warts, MC may appear and progress during pregnancy, and resolve spontaneously after delivery. Shared fomites can cause transmission and spread within the household and sporting venues.

The incubation period can vary from two weeks to six months. The typical lesions are pearly; umbilicated, multiple and measuring 2-4mm in diameter. The diagnosis is mostly clinical. Diagnosis on histology takes place when biopsy is performed on atypical lesions (e.g., after trauma, ulceration and/or secondary infection); or when there is medical uncertainty.

The MC lesions may resolve spontaneously within a few months. The lesions respond well to Podophyllotoxin (0.5% solution); which is practical for children and immuno-compromised patients, with multiple lesions. Cryo and electro-therapy is effective, but its application to multiple lesions is hindered by the impracticality of repeated and multiple applications. Imiquimod cream is effective and has a role in recurrent lesions. Following the early episodes of treatment, the patient should be warned that sub-clinical lesions could progress to apparent ones, within short period of treatment, which can cause disappointment and distress.

Chlamydia Trachomatis Genital Infections

The Organism

The Chlamydia trachomatis Species has four Biovars; two of which cause Chlamydial genital infections.

1. Lymphogranuloma venereum (LGV) Biovar; with three Serovars: L1, L2, L3.
2. Trachoma Biovar; with Serovars D-K causing Urethritis, Cervicitis, Salpingitis, Epididymitis, Proctitis, Conjunctivitis and Pneumonia of the newborn. Serovars A, B Ba, C cause Endemic Trachomal Conjunctivitis.

The Chlamydia trachomatis is an obligatory intracellular bacterium, wholly dependant on the host cell for energy and multiplication. The life cycle of the organism undergo tow phases, over 48-72hrs. The first is the Elementary Body, which infects columnar or pseudo-stratified columnar cells of the host and transform into the second phase, of a Reticulate Body (1μm). The later uses the host cell's nucleic acid to replicate and multiply for 24-48 hrs. It eventually produces elementary bodies, that burst out to re-infect other cells; and the cycle continues. Scientists have identified the nucleotide sequence of C trachomatis.

Infectivity and Transmission

The organism is transmitted by sexual intercourse. A single act of sexual intercourse, with an infected partner has a one in ten chance of transmission. Female patients are more vulnerable than the males in acquiring infections. The use of barrier contraception (e.g., a condom) reduces the possibility of transmission but does not eliminate the risk, due to accidents. Not every case of Chlamydial inoculation leads to progressive infection. Some infections, possibly one in five, end with spontaneous clearance. If un-treated, infection can persist for several years. The insidious nature of Chlamydia, the lack of symptoms in a proportion of patients and the long-term persistence of intra-cellular infection are leading causes for its transmission, propagation, spread and outbreaks.

Hand contamination with genital discharge may lead to conjunctival infection in adults. The Foetus may acquire the organism, during passage through an infected cervix/ genital tract; and develop conjunctivitis and /or pneumonia.

Prevalence

The WHO recognises Chlamydia trachomatis as a cause of more STDs than any other bacterial pathogen. Various studies estimate that 4-5 million ases of new genital Chlamydial infections take place in the USA, each year. The availability of specific mass investigative techniques (e.g., Nucleic Acid Amplification Techniques: NAATs) led to the identification of genital Chlamydial infection as the most common STI in the United Kingdom. The UK Health Protection Agency recorded over one hundred thousand new diagnosis of Chlamydia trachomatis, for year 2006, in GUM clinics; representing 166% increase from 1997. Studies calculate 1-4% prevalence in the UK general population; mounting to 5-15% in GUM and Family Planning Clinics. Multiplicity of sexual partners, short-term relationships, young age, and lack of consistent use of barrier contraception are observable risk factors. Females, between the age of 15 and 20, and males, between the age of 20 and 25, are most vulnerable. The Chlamydial infection rates, are in the region of 200 per 100,000 population in England, for males and females.

The lack of reliable investigations, in developing countries, undermines accurate diagnosis and epidemiological studies. There are no scientific reasons to presume that the condition is un-common in developing countries.

Clinical Presentation

The clinical features are variable; with up to 80% of females and 50% of males being asymptomatic. Men may act as disease carriers; spreading the condition, but rarely developing long term health problems. Infection could be silent for months or years; where the condition may be identified during a screening programme and/or routine testing. The general public awareness of sexual health issues brings patients to request tests "to exclude STIs"; and genital Chlamydia is the most commonly found one in the UK.

The immunological response, to chlamydial antigens, plays a significant role in the inflammatory process, increasing the risk of complications with repeated infections. Infections may persist for several years, leading to sub-acute and chronic chlamydial inflammatory process.

The first clinical presentation may be as early as seven days after the sexual contact that led to inoculation. Symptomatic patients may present with discharge (e.g., urethral or vaginal); and/or dysuria. Females may present with inter-menstrual and/or post-coital bleeding and/or menorrhagia and/or lower abdominal pain. The clinical findings of urethral discharge and/or meatitis in males; cervical inflammation, bleeding on touch, and/or mucopurulent cervicitis in females, should raise suspicion. The finding of White Blood Cells (WBCs) in the first catch urine test, WBCs on Gram stained /Microscopy read urethral smear in men gives supportive evidence for the diagnosis of urethritis. Chlamydia is the most common cause of Non- Gonococcal urethritis (NGU). The incidental finding of "cobble-stone" appearance on the cervix (e.g., during Colposcopic assessement for abnormal cervical cytology), should raise clinical suspicion. A positive NAAT should be ordered, to confirm or refute the diagnosis.

Chlamydial Proctitis could be silent, with no clinical symptoms or signs. It affects up to one in twenty females and one in ten homosexual males, attending GUM clinics. The covert infection and its possible asymptomatic nature, undermines its diagnosis; and therefore should be proactively excluded in patients giving history of receptive rectal sex. The finding of rectal inflammation, discharge and friability and/or a "cobble-stone" appearance, on on Proctoscopy, should raise clinical suspicion.

Neonatal Chllamydial Conjunctivitis is caused by acquisition from an infected cervical canal, during birth (*Vertical Transmission*). The Conjunctivitis usually present after leaving the post natal ward; therefore community practitioners are more likely to encounter the condition. Silent Chlamydial conjunctival infection may be diagnosed in a child up to several years, after delivery.

C trachomatis Conjunctivitis in adults is usually associated with genital Chlamydial infection. The modes of transmission to the conjuctival sac are accidental inoculation from an ejaculate and/or contaminated fingers (e.g., following foreplay). Adult Chlamydial Conjunctivitis in tropical and sub-tropical areas is an endemic condition, most likely due to the Trachoma biovars A, B, Ba and C.

Chlamydial pharyngeal infection may follow oral sex; and could be asymptomatic in many patients; to be found on investigations.

Pre-pubertal Chlamydial Vulvo Vaginitis should raise the question of child sexual abuse. Vertical transmission from mother to child can take place and may lie dormant. The identification of Chlamydial genital infection, beyond the age of three, should raise concerns of child sexual abuse. The immaturity of the vaginal epithelium in pre-pubertal girls makes it vulnerable to chlamydial infection.

Complications

Pelvic Inflammatory Disease (PID*)*, in variable degrees, is estimated to affect up to one in three female patients with untreated Genital Chlamydial infection. The sequellae of PID are menstrual irregularities, infertility, ectopic pregnancy and/or chronic pelvic pain. The long term consequences of PID require a proactive approach for early diagnosis and timely treatment of genital chlamydial infection. Ascending, Trans Cavity, Infection takes place through the cervical canal, uterine cavity, tubal lumen; then the peritoneal cavity. Lymphatic and haematogenous dissemination are known. Cervicitis, Endometritis, Salpingitis, Pelvic Peritonitis, upper abdominal Peritonitis and/or Peri-hepatitis (*Fitz-Hugh-Curtis Syndrome*) may occur in any combination.

Sexually Acquired Reactive Arthritis (SARA) is associated with genital chlamydial infection. *Reiter's Syndrome* is the combination of Poly-arthritis, Urethritis and/or Conjunctivitis.

C trachomatis organism has been identified in *Bartholin's abscess* and is a concomitant finding in male patients with *Epididymitis, Prostatitis and/or Seminal Vesiculitis.*

There is an association between Genital Chlamydial infection and *pre-term delivery, premature rupture of membranes and low birth weight.* Post-natally, it could lead to *Endometritis* and maternal pyrexia. Therapeutic Abortion, associated with untreated genital Chlamydia infection, may lead to PID. The clinical management of possible Chlamydial infections in relation to therapeutic abortion is dictated by clinical factors, local service and patient circumstances. Where there is certainty of patient's attendance for follow up, a Chlamydia test should be provided, followed by treatment of positive cases. Where follow up is not certain, there is a place for prophylactic therapy for Chlamydia, at the time of therapeutic abortion, due to the likelihood and seriousness of the complications, in the untreated case.

Neonatal Chlamydia infection may appear in the form of Conjunctivitis, Atypical pneumonia, Vaginitis, Pharyngitis and/or Otitis Media.

Investigations

The current laboratory investigatins for C trachomatis employ the Nucleic Acid Amplification Tests (NAAT) and DNA probes. The high specificity and sensitivity of the techniques improved detection rates; which contributed to the recent increase in diagnosis. NAAT lends itself to early detection, where a small dosage of organisms is identifiable, leading to a positive test result. The method is demanding on technology, staff and cost; which could be a hindrance in low cost health care settings. The NAAT are not approved by manufacturers for tests on rectal samples. The technology haven't been scrutinised for medico-legal purposes (e.g alleged rape). Cell culture remains the laboratory gold standard, with 100% specificity, therefore the method of choice in medico-legal cases. It requires expertise, which is not widely available.

The previous generation of Enzyme-linked Immuno-sorbent Assay (EIA), with its automated techniques for mass testing, reduced time and cost, and proved useful for clinical practice. Laboratories used "Direct Fluorescent Antibody" testing, as a supplementary method, to re-test samples reported positive by EIA, for confirmation.

Chlamydia serum antibody testing has no clinical value, except in supporting the diagnosis of neonatal pneumonia (i.e., raised Ig M) and scientific studies, where IgG indicates a past episodes of exposure and infection.

Treatment

Tetracyclines, Macrolides or Fluroquinolones provide alternative choices for the effective eradication of uncomplicated genital and/or rectal Chlamydia infections. Re-infection, from the same sex partner, can take place, if there is a time gape between treating sex contacts. Azithromycin (1g orally in a single dosage) is effective and convenient for the non-compliant patient. Doxycycline (100mg orally twice daily for seven days) is the option of first choice; but can lead to photosensitivity and the patient should be warned. Tetracycline (500mg orally four times daily for seven days) is a low-cost approach; but has compliance problems. Clarithromycin (400mg orally twice daily for seven days) or Ofloxacin (200mg orally twice daily for seven days) are suitable alternatives, but the higher cost is significant for large client base settings.

During pregnancy, Tetracyclines are contraindicated. Erythromycin (500mg orally four times daily, for seven days or 500mg twice daily for 14 days) had been used for pregnant patients. Gastrointestinal upsets tend to be prominent during pregnancy. Patient's compliance improves if they are fore-warned. Azithromycin is not licensed for use during pregnancy.

Failures in treatment are usually due to re-infection; following un-protected sexual intercourse with untreated partner. Treatment with Doxycycline or Azithromycin is effective. There are patients who express anxiety and request repeated treatment; possibly due to guilt feeling. They may present with symptoms; and tests in these cases are important, to provide objective assessment and avoid unnecessary repeat therapy. The absence of WBCs and/or Nitrates, in the first catch urine test, the absence of WBCs on urethral smear tests' Gram-staining and microscopy may call for NAAT. Repeat NAAT should be performed 3-4 weeks after treatment, to avoid the possibility of false positive results, with non-viable but detectable DNA strands. Negative tests provide the patient with the necessary assurance. A positive one suggests re-infection and requires re-treatment; and a repeated process of contact tracing.

Contact tracing and partner notification, client-led, provider-led, or a copbination of both, is an important part of the management and control of C trachomatis. Ideally, partner/s within several months of the diagnosis should be contacted and tested. Interpersonal and communication skills and expertise, plays an important role in contact tracing and health advising. Staff should gain patient's confidence and co-operation, to divulge sensitive information, regarding the patient and/or sex partner/s. Client-led contact tracing should be the first line of call, for its practicality. It can avoid un-necessary and avoidable communications and save   health care resources. The unit should make its expertise available to trace and contact the sex partner, if the patient is prepared to divulge information, but not willing to contact the partner, personally.

Gonorrhoea

Prevalence

Gonorrhoea is the second most commonly reported notifiable disease in the USA and the second most common bacterial STI in England and Wales. The WHO estimates that 62 million are infected with Gonorrhoea annually. The HPA recorded some 19,000 new cases of Gonorrhoea in UK for year 2006; 46% increase from 1997. During 2006 the burden of Gonorrhoea was high in young people; the highest in men aged 20-24 years (188/100,000 population) and women aged 16-19 years (128/100,000 population). Between 1996 and 2006, the diagnosis of gonorrhoea in men has risen by 30%; compared to 152% for homosexually acquired infections, which also accounts for 1/3 of all diagnosed cases.

The incidence of Gonorrhoea varies between different communities and periods. The prevalence reflects public knowledge, anxiety of STIs, testing for other STIs (eg. Chlamydia), the use of barrier contraception methods and/or patterns of antibiotic use in the community, leading to the incidental treatment of a concurrent gonorrheal infection. Certain socio- demographic factors increase patients' vulnerability. Risk factors are young age, urbanisation, lower socio-economic standards, social instability and/or ethnic minority status. Public Health Organisations follow up gonorrhoea, as a surrogate marker for casual, unsafe and high risk sexual practices.

The Organism

The causative organism is Neisseria gonorrhoeae; a Gram negative diplococcous. The organism is distinguished, from other Neisseria species, by specific serological reactions; which subgroup the gonococcal strain. This is subdivided into serovars, according to the subtypes of gonococcal outer-membrane proteins. Scientists have identified the nucleotide sequence of N gonorrhoeae

Transmission

N gonorrhoeae is vulnerable to dryness and temperature; therefore requires intimate contact for transmission (i.e sexual intercourse). It infects the columnar epithelium of the lower genital tract, rectum and/or pharynx. Females are more susceptible than males in acquiring the infection, following a single episode of sexual intercourse. Sexual transmission is the most likely route of acquisition. Non-sexual transmission (i.e by fomites) is theoretically possible, but very unlikely; due to the natural vulnerability of the organism to temperature, desiccation and oxygen. Direct inoculation is possible (e.g., Sharing sex toys and/or the immediate direct inoculation by fingers, following foreplay).

The organism adheres first to the epithelial cells, infects the epithelial layer then penetrates into the sub-epithelial space, initiating the inflammatory process and its complications. Trans-luminal spread in males can lead to Prostatitis and in females leads to PID and peritonitis. Haematogenous and lymphatic spread is thought to take place in 1% of cases, leading to Disseminated Gonococcal Infections (eg. Arthritis). Some infections eventually clear spontaneously. Most pharyngeal infections clear within three months but data on the clearance of ano-genital disease are not available.

Clinical Presentation

The clinical picture depends on the susceptibility of the individual host, affected site, virulence and innoculum of the organism. The incubation period varies from 1-14 days. Males usually present with profuse discharge and/or Dysuria. One in ten males could be asymptomatic, to be diagnosed on routine testing and/or contact tracing. The proportion of asymptomatic females is higher, reaching 70%. Females present usually with vaginal discharge. The clinical finding of muco-purulent, urethral or cervical, discharge during routine examination should raise suspicion. The findings may not be typical in early or less severe cases. The signs may be as little as inflammation of the urethral meatus (Meatitis). Gonorrhoeal infection should be excluded pro-actively, in young females presenting with lower abdominal pain and significant sexual history.

Gonorrhoeal Proctitis affects mainly homosexual men and is a surrogate marker of high-risk sexual activity of the index case and/or partner/s. It is asymptomatic in most of the cases. It may present with discharge, pain and/or rectal bleeding. There may be evidence of inflammation on rectal examination and proctoscopy. The attending clinician should encourage the patient to give accurate sexual history, to identify the sites necessary for examination, and collection of samples for tests and swabs, with an informed consent. Rectal examination in a patient that denies rectal intercourse or symptoms could be questionable. It would tantamount to medical negligence to overlook rectal examination in a patient who presents with history of rectal sex and/or symptoms.

Gonorrhoeal pharyngitis could be asymptomatic in most of the patients; therefore pharyngeal swabs are indicated for patients giving history of oral sex. Pharyngeal infection requires a longer period of treatment and carries the additional risk of dissemination; therefore it is important to make the diagnosis or excluding it; even in the presence of concurrent urethritis or cervicitis.

Gonococcal conjunctivitis is a serious condition that can lead to keratitis and blindness. The condition is not common in adults. In a neo-nate, it indicates vertical transmission. The mother and her sex partner, in this case, require assessment, investigations and treatment.

The non-sexual transmission of gonorrhoea to pre-pubertal children is possible but not likely; due to the natural vulnerability of the organism. The attending clinician should consider the possibility of child sexual abuse.

Gonococcal infection may spread through the male urethra into the surrounding para-urethral glands, leading to abscess and/or cellulitis; eventually leading to urethral strictures and fistulae. Trans-luminal spread can take place into the bulbo-urethral glands, prostate, seminal vesicles and epididymis; leading to cascades of inflammations (e.g., Prostatitis, Seminal Vesiculitis and/or Epididymitis). The clinical presentation depends on the site and extent of inflammation (e.g., Pain during erection, ejaculation, micturition and/or defecation). Tenderness at the site of the inflammation depends on the extent of spread and could be localised or generalized.

Pelvic Inflammatory Disease is thought to affect one in five women who remain untreated for gonorrhoea. The condition may be a range of Endometritis, Salpingitis, Oopheritis, Peritonitis, and/or Peri-hepatitis (*Fitz Hugh-Curtis Syndrome*). The organism can cause Bartholin's abscesses and can lead to inflammation of the para-urethral glands.

The *Disseminated Gonococcal Infection (DGI)* is becoming less common due to better diagnosis, earlier treatment and wider use of antibiotic therapy. The use of antibiotics, for a non-related/non gonococcal infection, may incidentally treat a concurrent un-diagnosed gonococcal infection. The cumulative effect is a reduction in DGI. Predisposing factors for DGI include pharyngeal infection, pregnancy and peri-menstrual inoculation of N gonorrhoeae. Some sub-groups of N gonorrhoeae are more likely to cause DGI. The patient usually presents with a skin rash, arthritis and mild pyrexia. The typical skin lesion is necrotic pustules; but may present with petechiae or papules. The affected joints may be single or multiple, small or large and migratory. The spread may cause hepatitis, meningitis and/or endo/peri/myo/carditis.

Gonorrhoea during pregnancy may lead to early gestational loss, sceptic abortion and/or PID. Later in pregnancy, it may lead to chorio-amnionitis, premature rupture of membranes, pre-term delivery and/or low birth weight. In the post natal maternal pyrexia, Gonorrhoea, should be part of the differential diagnosis and proactively excluded, especially in a patient with any of the risk factors.

Ophthalmia Neonatorum is less common than it used to be in developed countries. The infection usually presents within few days of delivery with profuse discharge. The condition is serious and may lead to Keratitis, Ulceration, Pan-ophthalmitis and blindness. Neo-natal prophylactic installation of anti-gonococcal eye drops is practiced in communities where there is a chance of undiagnosed maternal gonorrhoea. The installation of 1% Silver Nitrate solution, in the conjuctival sac of at risk newborns, is of value in low cost settings. Alternatively, 1% Tetracycline or 0.5% Erythromycin ointment provide prophylaxis in most cases.

Maternal gonorrhoea may contaminate other mucosal orifices in the newborn, leading to Pharyngitis, Rhinitis, Vaginitis, Urethritis, and/or Proctitis. Systemic spread may lead to arthritis and/or meningitis.

Diagnosis

Urethral, cervical, pharyngeal and/or rectal swabs, for microbiological culture and antibiotic susebtibility tests are necessary for management. GUM clinics in UK have facilities for on-site Gram staining and microscopy reading; where the organism will be identified as Gram Negative Intracellular Diplococci (GNDC). The microscopy test can identify up to 90% of male urethritis. In females, the test is less sensitive and can identify one in two infected females. The Gram staining and microscopy tests allow the early initiation of treatment, advice regarding abstinence from sex, barrier protection and contact tracing. Other forms of pharyngeal Neisserial commensals interferes with the test's validity; therefore microscopy is not suitable for diagnosing pharyngeal gonorrhoea. Direct inoculation of the organism into a culture medium and immediate incubation is preferable. Alternatively, a special transport medium and timely transfer to laboratory is required. The arrangements should be well planned between the clinician and recipient microbiology laboratory. NAAT for N gonorrhoeae could be done in parallel with that for C trachomatis. Traditional cultures still provide the benefit of antibiotics susceptibility, which is essential for treatment. The organism is notorious of changing its susceptibility to antibiotics; and therefore it is prudent to base treatment on sensitivity tests.

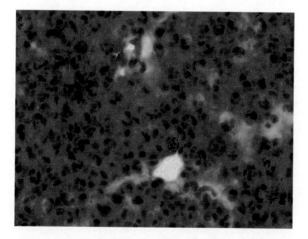

Figure 1. Gram-stained Microscopy slide showing PMN in case of Cervicitis

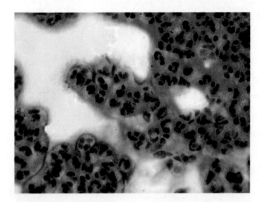

Figure 2. Gram-stained Microscopy slide showing GNID

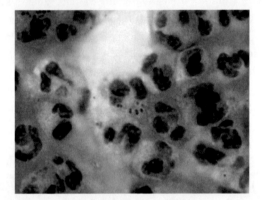

Figure 3. Gram-stained Microscopy slide showing GNID

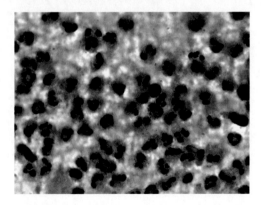

Figure 4. Gram-stained Microscopy slide showing PMN in case of Urithritis

Treatment

Antibiotic resistance causes a clinical problem, with patients receiving inadequate, improper, or ineffective antibiotics, counterfeit medicines and/or sub-standard dosages.

The recommended therapy, prior to sensitivity tests, is either Ceftriaxone (250mg IM)[125mg according to USA-CDC], or Cefixime (400mg oral). In patients with penicillin allergy, Spectinomycin (2g IM) or Azithromycin (1g oral) are useful alternatives. The widespread use of Azithromycin could lead to rapid emergence of resistance; therefore should be rationalised. Alternative regimes are Ciprofloxacin (500mg oral), Ofloxacin (400mg oral) or Ampicilline (2gm + Probenecid 1gm oral).

Disseminated Gonococcal Infection (DGI) requires hospitalisation and parenteral therapy. The initial regimen is Ceftriaxone (1gm, IM or IV, every 24 hours), Cefotaxine (1gm, IV, every eight hours) or Spectinomycin (2gm, IM, every 12 hours). The parenteral regime is then followed by an oral therapy, after clinical improvement: Cefixime (400mg orally BD) or Ofloxacin (400mg, BD, for 7 days). Fluroquinolones could be an alternative, if the antimicrobial susceptibility is confirmed.

Clinical Practicalities

1. The diagnosis of GNID on microscopy should lead to the initiation of antibiotic therapy, that is effective against gonorrhoea, for urethritis and/or cervicitis. It is wise not to base the diagnosis of gonorrhoea, on microscopy alone, without the result of culture tests. The incidental demise of the organism, during transport or culture, could lead to avoidable distress.

2. A "test of cure" was traditionally performed but no longer required; when treatment is based on antibiotic susceptibility studies.

3. There could be a clinical place, in some conditions, for A Test of "Compliance", to ascertain the patient's compliance with the clinical advice (i.e., to abstain from sexual intercourse, until both partners complete treatment).

4. Contact tracing of partner/s, investigations to exclude other STIs, epidemiological treatment for concurrent Chlamydia and tracing of the

transmission chains or clusters, should be initiated as soon as practically possible.

5. Gonorrhoea is encountered frequently in men having sex with men (MSM). It could be used as a surrogate marker of high risk sexual activity.

6. Pharyngeal gonorrhoea require longer period of therapy; therefore its concurrent identification, or exclusion, is clinically indicated.

7. New patterns of antibiotic resistance are continiously emerging. Both clinicians and microbiologists should be vigilant.

8. DNA typing of the N gonorrhoeae organism, with Plasmids / DNA fragments, could be of value for forensic cases.

9. Sero, Auxo and/or Opa-typing are of epidemiological value; for contact tracing studies and research of cluster cases.

Non-Specific Urethritis

Non-Specific Urethritis (NSU) is a diagnosis that is reached following the exclusion of infections with C.trachomatis and/or N.gonorrhoea, as an underlying cause of the Urethritis. The condition of Urethritis is diagnosed first on clinical grounds (i.e., dysuria and discharge), the presence of WBCs in the First Catch Urine (FCU) and WBCs on microscopic examination of Gram stained urethral smear or sediments from FCU.

The Gram stained urethral smear preparation show Polymorph Nuclear Leucocytes (PMNLs) on high powe field (HPF) microscopic examination. PMNLs of 5-10 or more/HPF; with the repeated findings in five fields, is considered as evidence of urethritis. The Dip stick urine test can identify WBCs in urine. It can also identify Nitrates, as indirect evidence of WBCs.

NSU is multi-factorial. Sexual acquisition is widely accepted the main contributing factor. There could be clinical and microscopic evidence of urethritis in a patient without any symptoms. The patient complains of urethral discharge, Dysuria, urethral discomfort and/or frequency of micturition. On genital examination, there may be urethral discharge (Mucoid, Purulent or Mucopurulent), Meatal inflammation (Meatitis) and/or Peri-meatitis. The urethritis could be part of Balano-posthitis.

Causation

Non Gonococcal Urethritis (NGU), is the temporary diagnosis in a patient identified with urethtritis and in the absence of GNID on microscopic examination of the Gram-stained urethral smear. Clinical facilities that have the benefits and skills for on-site Gram staining and microscopic examination, should have the capacity for the accurate identification of GNID, in 90% of cases, if N gonorrhoea is the underlying cause. Some 20-30% of conditions initially identified as NGU would later report positive for C.trachomatis. If tests for both N.gonorrhoea and C.trachomatis are negative, then the condition is non-Gonococcal, non-Chlamydial Urethritis; or Non-Specific Urethritis (NSU).

1. Recent studies suggested some 20% of patients presenting with symptomatic urethritis had C trachomatis, some 10% Mycloplasma genitalium and no detectable pathogen in some 70%.
2. Males practising insertive anal sex may have NSU associated with Coliform bacteria.
3. Ureaplasma urealyticum may be associated with NSU, but its rule as a causative agent is not clear, as there are conflicting research findings.
4. Herpes simplex may cause urethral ulceration and consequently inflammation and urethritis.
5. Candidal urethritis may be part of Balanoposthitis.

Treatment

GUM clinics start antibiotic treatment at the initial clinical and microscopic confirmation of Urethritis. The antibiotic therapy should cover the possibilities of both C.trachomatis and/or N.gonorrhoea. The antibiotic susceptibility and resistance patterns for N gonorrhoea should be considered in prescribing therapy. Doxycycline (100mg, orally, twice daily, for 7 days) or Azithromycin (1gm, orally, single dose) is the recommended first-line treatment regimen. Alternative regimens include: Tetracycline (500mg, orally, 4 times daily, for 7 days), Minocycline (100mg, orally, once daily, for 7 days), Erythromycin (500mg, orally, twice daily, for 14 days) or Ofloxacin (200mg, orally, twice daily or 400mg, once daily, for 7 days).

Practical Considerations

1. The initial diagnosis is one of Urethritis, which carries the possibility of being Chlamydial and/or Gonococcal in origin. For this reason the prescribed treatment should cover both organisms.

2. The patient is advised to abstain from sexual intercourse, till both partners are investigated and treated.

3. The sex partner/s require assessment and investigations.

4. There is conflicting evidence regarding the benefit of prescribing treatment to female partners of NSU patients (i.e., epidemiological treatment for NSU contacts). There have been reports of patients with persistent and/or recurrent urethritis, being cured only after the treatment of the sex partner/s. Mycoplasma genitalium accounts for some 20% of NSU cases and probably contributes to female pelvic infections, which provide grounds for the epidemiological treatment of NSU contacts

5. Understandably, female partners with evidence of N.gonorrohea, C.trachomatis, Trichomonas vaginalis infection and/or Bacterial vaginosis would require treatment accordingly. The female patient's test results are usually available after that of her male partner and both test results should be cross-referred.

6. There is evidence that suggests an association between asymptomatic NSU and Bacterial vaginosis in the female sex partner.

7. The identification of female partner's infections may have a bearing on the treatment of the male NSU (e.g., Trichomoniasis and/or Vulvo Vaginal Candidiasis).

8. Both partners should be advised to abstain from sexual intercourse, until their investigations are fulfilled and the treatment course is completed.

9. A short course of treatment with azithromycin have lead some patients to resume intercourse early. Abstinence and barrier contraception's, for two week interval, should be advisable after the initiation of treatment.

10. Antibiotics routinely prescribed for Chlamydial and Gonococcal Urethritis have anti-inflammatory effect, which would help in combating the Urethritis

11. Male patients should be encouraged to abandon any urethral self-examination, which may provoke or prolong the urethritis.

Resistant, Recurrent and Chronic NSU

One patient in five, may suffer persistent urethritis, despite treatment and in the clear absence of re-infection. There is a challenge in making the diagnosis (that sexual intercourse and re-infection did not take place). If the condition persist beyond four weeks, it is considered ChronicNSU. The rule of Ureaplasma urealyeicum and/or Mycoplasma genitalium in recurrent and chronic NSU is considered but not fully elucidated. The role of organisms in partner's developing PID is attracting increasing recognition and concern. There are clinical grounds in the treatment of persistent and chronic NSU. It addresses the male patient's symptoms; and avoid the chance of PID in the female partner. Erythromycin (500mg, orally, 4 times daily, for two weeks) plus Metronidazole (400mg, orally, twice daily, for 5 days) is the recommended treatment of choice. The female partner should receive epidemiological treatment with Erythromycin.

Practical Considerations

1. Some patients will continue to complain of symptoms of urethritis, have discharge and show evidence of PMNSs on urethral smear and microscopy and/or evidence of WBCs in the (FCU).
2. There should be a clinical, microscopic and urinary findings to reach the diagnosis. There are patients who are worried and request tests for further assurance. This was perpetuated by the past GUM practice of "Tests of Cure".
3. The clinician should proactively consider and exclude the possibility of concomitant urinary tract infections and/or Prostatitis. There should be a differential diagnosis with urinary tract infections, bacterial and non-bacterial prostatitis, before concluding recurrent NSU.
4. The underlying cause could be incomplete treatment and/or unprotected sexual intercourse with an infected/untreated partner (i.e., new acquisition); rather than persistent or recurrent urethritis. It is important to establish that the patient completed his initial course of treatment and did not have unprotected intercourse.
5. It is prudent to exclude chemical and/or traumatic urethritis, before assuming recurrent or persistent NSU. Materials excreted in urine (e.g., alcohol) may cause of urethral irritation and inflammation. Traumatic irritation of the urethra (e.g., vigorous masturbation) can lead to the urethral inflammation. There is paucity in clinical research in the area of chemical and traumatic urethritis.and neither conditions had the benefits of scientific studies.

Muco-Purulent Cervicitis

Mucopurulent cervicitis (MPC) is a clinical entity identified with evidence of mucopurulent discharge and cervical inflammation. Severe MPC is associated with greenish-yellowish cervical mucopurulent discharge, cervical swelling, hyperaemia, oedema, and/or ectopy. In less developed MPC, the discharge is evident on swabbing the cervical canal with cotton-tipped swab (swab test), which may also provoke persistent bleeding. In mild cases of MPC, the patients are usually asymptomatic or may have non specific symptoms (e.g., Inter-Menstrual Bleeding (IMB) and/or Post Coital Bleeding (PCB), which may be the first finding to attract the patient's attention. In severe cases, excessive vaginal discharge may be the main presentation. The presence of PMNLs on Gram-stained endocervical smear and microscopy test is non-specific and should not be used to support or exclude the diagnosis of MPC. The presence of leucorrhoea, > 10 WBCs/HPF, on microscopic examination of vaginal fluid in the absence of inflammatory vaginitis, have some sensitive indication of cervicitis. The test has high negative value.

Causation

1. C trachomatis and/or N gonorrhoea are leading causes of cervicitis. Non-specific cervicitis is identified in the absence of the two organisms.
2. Cervicitis could be associated with Herpetic cervical lesions and the patient may not have an associated vulval HSV lesion.
3. The role of M genitalium and BV suggests association, but no evidence of direct causation, with MPC.

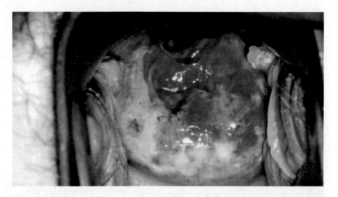

Figure 1. Cervicitis

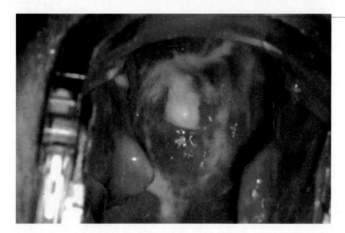

Figure 2. Muco-Purulent Cervicitis

Treatment

Clinical evidence of cervicitis gives ground for the initiation of empirical antibiotic therapy; with a spectrum of cover for C trachomatis and N gonorrhoea. Azithromycin (1g orally in a single dose), or Doxycycline (100 mg orally twice a day for 7 days). Evidence of associated T vaginalis or BV would call for the addition of Metronidazole (400 mg twice daily for 7 days).

There are benefits in cryotherapy for cervical ectopy associated with MPC. The presence of large cervical ectopy (i.e., eversion of the endocervical columnar epithelium to replace the stratified epithelium of the ectocervix) increases the chances for cervicitis. The columnar epithelium of the cervical canal, have the capacity to harbour organisms, which promotes Cervicitis. Cryotherapy will cause necrosis of the columnar epithelium and give an opportunity for the stratified epithelium to resurface the ectocervix. Cervical electro-cauterisation was used in the past for the treatment of severe mucopurulent cervicitis. There have been cases of cervical cicatrisation, following electro-cautery to the cervix. If severe, the cicatrisation can interfere with cervical dilatation during labour; therefore cervical cauterization should be avoided.

Practical Considerations

1. Male partners of patients identified with MPC caused by C trachomatis or N gonorrhoea should be traced for investigations and treatment.
2. Many cases of clinically diagnosed MPC may prove negative for organisms, but still worthy of treatment of the patient and partner.
3. The role of Mycoplasma and Ureaplasma in MPC is still under scrutiny.
4. It would be wise to initiate treatment of the partner, for the corresponding infections and advise both partners to abstain from sexual intercourse for at least a week, from the time of the last treated partner.

Pelvic Inflammatory Disease

Pelvic Inflammatory Disease (PID) is inflammation of the female genital tract; and may include any or all of the following: Endometritis, Salpingitis, Oophoritis, Parametritis and/or pelvic peritonitis. The female genital tract has elaborate protective mechanisms; that counteract infection and inflammation. The defensive mechanisms include the vaginal-floral balance, cervical mucus plug, cellular and humoral immune mechanisms. The loss in balance of these mechanisms predisposes to PID. Vaginal colonisation with organisms, their access through the cervical canal, the presence of menstrual blood and/or endometrial debris in the uterine cavity, the opening of the fallopian tubes into the peritoneal cavity and the ability of some organisms to travel with spermatozoae, make women vulnerable to ascending genital tract infections. The spread of infection is usually ascending, through cervical, uterine cavity and fallopian tubes. The spread may be trans-peritoneal from an adjacent inflamed organ (e.g., Appendicitis), haematogenous or lymphatic (e.g., E coli, from urinary tract). A collection of puss may lead to pelvic abscess (e.g., Abscess of Pouch of Douglas), salpingo-ovarian abscess or uterine abscess. The latter may affect elderly patients, who suffer post-menopausal genital tract atrophy and cervical stenosis.

The average annual incidence of PID, in females aged 15-24 in western countries, is 2 per thousand. In the USA, it is estimated that annually, more than 1,000,000 women experience an episode of acute PID and 100,000 become infertile as a result of PID.

Women are vulnerable to PID during menstruation, following instrumentation (e.g., termination of pregnancy) and pregnancy. A previous episode of PID increases the woman's risk to subsequent episodes. Age represents a relative risk factor. The under-25 years are at more risk of developing PID; due to their vulnerability to STIs. The exposure of a woman to multiple sex partners; and a woman whose partner has more than one sex partner, have an increased chance of exposure to STIs consequently at risk of PID. Vaginal douching is not a common practice in the UK; but is widespread in different cultures. Douching can disturb the vaginal ph and floral balance, facilitate the ascent of organism through the cervical canal with the fluid jet and encouraging PID. Intrauterine Device (IUD) insertion may increase the risk of PID; but patient selection and the prior testing for STIs, reduces the risk.

The use of barrier contraception (e.g., condoms, diaphragms and spermicides) reduce the risk of PID. The oral contraceptive pill, especially the Progesterone only pill, enhances the cervical mucus plug and reduces the risk of PID. The seriousness of pregnancy associated infections requires additional clinical vigilance, if-ante-natal pelvic infection is suspected. Pregnancy associated thickening of the cervical mucus plug reduces the risk of PID, but does not eliminate its chances.

Sexually transmitted infections, were identified in different percentages of patients diagnosed with PID, according to the study population. N gonorrhoea and C trachomatis were found in 1:2 to 1:20 in PID patients. There is an increasing perception in the medical community that past estimates of untreated N gonorroea and C trachomatis, leading to the acquisition of PID, were over emphasised. In the past, up to 30% of untreated cervical Chlamydial or Gonococcal infections were thought to lead to PID, but this percentage is the subject of recent debates. The long-term consequences of PID are significant and include infertility, ectopic pregnancy and/or chronic pelvic pain.

There is a statistically significant association between Bacterial Vaginosis (BV) and PID. The recovery of organisms associated with BV from the endometrium and fallopian tubes in cases of PID, support the observation. Bacterial enzymes, Sialidase from Bacteroides and Prevotella species, lead to changes in the cervical mucus, reduce its protective capacity and predispose to PID.

Other organisms that have been recovered in association with PID include: Streptococci (group A-D and Viridans), Escherichia coli, Staphylococci (Coagulase negative), Mycoplasma genitalium and hominis and Actinomyces israelii (in association with IUDs). Rarely PID could be a part of a generalised specific abdominal infection/ inflammation (e.g., Tuberculosis, Typhoid and Paratyphoid).

Clinical Presentation

Sexual health awareness has initiated an increasing number of patients to request tests, to exclude STIs. This lead to the early identification and treatment of infections at a pre-clinical stage. This may have influenced the decline in the incidence of Gonnococcal and/or Chlamydial PID. The availability of health care resources opens the opportunity of diagnosis and treatment of PID, at an early stage; well before a full-blown and typical clinical picture.

The typical presentation of acute PID is acute pelvic/ lower abdominal pain, deep Dyspareunia and vaginal discharge. In severe conditions, the patients may have nausea and vomiting. Peri-menstrual episodes may present with irregular vaginal-bleeding and Dysmenorrhea. Pyrexia ($>38^0$C), is likely in severe cases. A false low temperature reading may be caused by the intake of over-the-counter analgesics/antipyretics. The patient may have any or all of the following signs: lower abdominal pain and tenderness, with guarding and rebound, deep pelvic pain and tenderness on vaginal bimanual examination and tenderness on moving a cervix and/or adenexae (cervical excitation). Where clinical care is accessible, the finding of pelvic mass (e.g., Tupo-ovarian abscess), have reduced, following early diagnosis and treatment of PID. Severe PID, and/or delayed treatment, may progress to generalised peritonitis, paralytic ileus and abdominal distension.

A woman presenting with lower abdominal-pelvic pain and tenderness with cervical excitation, should be proactively managed, with PID at the top of the list of differential diagnosis.

Complications

Chronic PID may be clinically silent or present with constant or intermittent lower abdominal pain, Dyspareunia, backache and/or menstrual irregularities. In recurrent cases, progressive pelvic adhesions may take place and lead to distortions in pelvic anatomy. Inflamation from right Salpingo-oophoritis may spread to the peri-appendicular peritoneum and mimic appendicitis. Progressive inflammation may lead to tubo-ovarian- appendiceal mass.

Recurrent episodes of PID may lead to permanent tubal damage and infertility. Milder episodes of PID may damage tubal epithelial functions, leading to patent but dysfunctional tubes. Progressive PID lead to tubal occlusion, collection of fluid (Salpingo- coele), peri-tubal adhesions and distortion. The patient may present with infertility and PID is incidentally found during laparoscopic investigations. If conception takes place following tubal damage and adhesions, it carries the risk of ectopic pregnancy. Pelvic adhesions and interstitial inflammation, are associated with recurrent episodes of Pelvic Pain, Dysmenorrhoea and/or Dyspareunia.This can reduces the quality of life and lead to psycho-social and psycho-sexual difficulties. Fitz-Hugh-Curtis Syndrome described perihepatitis, which is a consequence of trans-peritoneal and lymphatic spread. The patient may present with abdominal right upper quadrant pain, radiating to shoulder, worsening with inspiration and movement. There may be tenderness in the right upper quadrant and positive Murphy's sign (i.e., pain associated with palpation below the right costal margin and deep inspiration). The patient may or may not have other clinical evidence of PID. The condition requires a differential diagnosis with consideration of inflammatory conditions of the gall bladder, right lower lung and/or pleural lobes; and more seriously, pulmonary embolism.

Investigations

Young women presenting with lower abdominal pain should undergo proactive methodological clinical assessment, that includes PID, for differential diagnosis. If the clinician considered other diagnoses, PID should be proactively excluded due to the seriousness of its consequences (e.g., infertility, ectopic pregnancy and/or chronic pelvic pain).

Cervical, vaginal and/or urethral, swabs should be taken, with special reference to N gonorrhoea, C trachomatis and Anaerobes. The presence of Polymorph Nuclear Leucocytes (PMNLs) is a frequent finding in Gram- stained cervical smears and may not be associated with a clinically identifiable PID. PMNLs are less likely to be absent in a clinically identified case of PID (i.e., high negative predictive value).

Microbiological investigations, culture and antibiotic suseptibility tests are routeinly ordered. They should include tests for N gonorrhoeae and C trachomatis. The management and antibiotic therapy usually start on clinical grounds, empirical basis and prior to obtaining the microbiology results.

A high Erythrocyte Sedimentation Rate (ESR) and C-Reactive Protein (CRP) are supportive of an inflammatory process that could be due to PID. The tests may only be found in three-quarters of cases. The presence of elevated ESR/CRP, WBCs in blood and/or PMNLs in aGram-stained cervical smear should support the diagnosis of PID; but their absence does not exclude PID.

The clinician should request abdominal and pelvic ultra-sonography (US), as part of the process of differential diagnosis, which is helpful when abortion or ectopic pregnancy is considered. It could also help or exclude the diagnosis of PID associated pelvic mass/abscess (e.g., tubo-ovarian mass). A negative ultrasonic finding does not exclude the diagnosis of PID.

Laparoscopy is invasive procedure and should be considered on the balance of its risk, complications and/or availability of resources. The case for laparoscopy is stronger, when a differential diagnosis between PID and ectopic pregnancy may not be possible on clinical deductions. The availability of high sensitivity β Human Chrionic Gonadotrophins (β HCG) tests and high definition ultra-sonography, have increased the accuracy of diagnosis of ectopic pregnancy. The need of emergency laparoscopy, for the diagnosis of ectopic pregnancy is declining. There continues to be a place for laparoscopy in the diagnosis of chronic and silent PID, where the woman's main complaint is "lower abdominal/pelvic pain of unknown origin". Laparoscopy could help to identify the aetiology of the lower abdominal pain (e.g., endometriosis, pelvic adhesions); or exclude it. The laparoscopic findings of tubal oedema, hyperaemia, exudate and/or adhesions, support the diagnosis of acute/sub-acute PID. In chronic PID, the finding may be a range of mild peri-tubal and pelvic adhesions, distortion, amalgamation of pelvic organs and /or peri-hepatic adhesions.

Endometrial samples, for histology and microbiological investigations, could support the clinical diagnosis; but are mostly used for research. The invasive nature of the test, the risk of breaching the natural defence barriers and the time interval between the clinical presentation and availability of results, make it impractical to wait for its results prior to the initiation of therapy.

Differential Diagnosis

The process of clinical assessment for suspected PID should be a methodological process of differential diagnosis. The lack of specificity and sensitivity, of the signs, symptoms and investigations, requires a low threshold for clinical suspicion. Acute appendicitis, ectopic pregnancy, rupture or torsion of ovarian cyst, acute urinary tract infections and other causes of acute abdomen should be considered in the differential diagnosis of PID. The consequences of a misdiagnosed case of PID or ectopic pregnancy are serious and either conditions should be proactively excluded in acute pelvic/ lower abdominal pain.

In chronic PID, the differential diagnosis includes endometriosis, rupture or torsion of ovarian cyst, intestinal inflammation and upper/lower urinary tract infection. The similarities of recurrent chronic PID and endometriosis, where both lead to pelvic adhesions, distortions and amalgamations; require a definitive diagnosis in patients presenting with "chronic pelvic pain". Laparoscopy could define the underlying cause and direct selective therapy. There have been medico-legal cases brought against clinicians on the grounds of failing to proactively consider, diagnose, treat or exclude PID, in women presenting with lower abdominal pain, when the condition was later found on laparoscopic investigation.

Clinical Practicalities

1. No single medical history, clinical examination or laboratory finding can detect all cases of PID or exclude all women without PID (i.e., the diagnostic criteria lack both sensitivity and specificity).
2. In view of the serious consequences of PID, there should be a low threshold for clinical suspension, diagnosis and start of empirical treatment. The minimal criteria of uterine/adnexal tenderness and/or cervical motion tenderness should bring a provisional diagnosis.
3. A patient who was diagnosed with mild PID and commenced on oral therapy should have the opportunity of a clinical review, if the condition worsen or does not improve.
4. A patient with severe PID, who is managed with oral therapy, should have a clinical review following 3 days of treatment to ensure improvement; otherwise revision of therapy, including hospitalisation and parenteral treatment, should be considered.
5. Doxycycline does not cover Streptococcous viridans, Coliforms and some strains of N gonorrhoea developed resistance to it.
6. Mycoplasma hominis and Ureaplasma urealyticum may cause PID in some cases; and should be considered in the choice of antibiotic therapy.

Management of PID

Antibiotic treatment should be started early on the grounds of clinical diagnosis, as delay could leads to long term complications. In-patient care is indicated in severe PID or systemic effects; when parenteral treatment is deemed necessary. When the patient presents with acute abdomen, there is a case for further investigations, to exclude other gynaecological or surgical emergencies (e.g., appendicitis, ectopic pregnancy, pelvic or tubo-ovarian abscess). Awating the result should not delay the start of antibiotics, which could be reviewed at a later stage.

The patient's general condition dictates the need for bed rest, which include abstinence from sexual intercourse. The sex partner should be adviced on investigations to exclude STIs. There is a case for offering him epidemiological treatment; as some of organisms are not routinely investigated (e.g., Mycoplasma hominis and genitalium). The patient requires two weeks of continuous antibiotic therapy. In severe PID, parenteral treatment should be started first. The regimen should include anti-microbial against C Trachomatis, N Gonorrhoeae and Anaerobes.

The initial parenteral regimens may be a choice of Ceftriaxone (250 mg, stat, IM) or Cefoxitin (2 g, stat, IM) plus Probenecid (1 g oral) or Cefoxitin (2 g, TID, IV) plus Doxycycline (100 mg, BD, IV) or Clindamycin (900 mg, TID, IV) plus Gentamicin (2 mg/kg of body weight loading dose, IV or IM; followed by 1.5 mg/kg TID).

The parenteral therapy should be continued for 24 hours after clinical improvement. Oral therapy should target a spectrum for Gram-negative facultative bacteria and Streptococci (e.g., Doxycycline, 100 mg, BD, orally and Metronidazole 400mg, BD, orally), to complete two weeks of treatment.

In mild/ moderate PID, the out-patient treatment should follow similar principles of compination therapy for a period of two weeks. Ofloxacin (400 mg, orally, BD) and Metronidazole (400 mg, orally, BD) provide alternative to Doxycycline/Metronidazole.

Special Situations

1. When Tubo-ovarian abscess is diagnosed, Clindamycin (450 mg orally 4 times a day) or Metronidazole (400 mg orally 4 times a day) is indicated, to extend the spectrum of treatment to Anaerobic infections.
2. Ofloxacin was considered in combination therapy, but the lack of coverage for Anaerobic infections raises concern.
3. Amoxycillin/Clavulanic Acid plus Doxycycline are notorious of gastrointestinal symptoms and can leads to patient compliance problems.

4. PID with pregnancy is a high-risk situation which is associated with maternal and foetal morbidity, foetal demise or preterm delivery. Hospitalisation and parenteral antibiotics should be commenced as soon as possible.

5. Doxycycline is contra-indicated during pregnancy and should be replaced with Erythromycin (50 mg/kg, IV,daily).

6. HIV patient developing PID carries an increased risk; which is higher at the later stage of immuno-compromise. The patient is more likely to have tubo-ovarian abscesses, higher rate of concomitant infections with M.hominis, Candida and Streptococcal infections.

7. PID in immuno-deficient HIV patients requires hospitalisation and parenteral treatment but the response is good to standard antibiotics.

Prevention

Sexual health education is viewed as a positive step towards prevention of STIs and their complications. Supportive evidence is drawn from comparative analysis of rates of conditions in countries/states that apply education with those who do not. Theoretically, the use of barrier contraception should give some protection from STIs and their complications. Contact tracing aim to identify patients and partners, who are at risk of complications and/or act as reservoirs for infections.

The National Chlamydia Screening programs are hypothesised to reduce the incidence of PID. Patient awareness of STIs consequences and early attendance to seek medical advice reflects on early diagnosis and treatment, which circumvent STIs and their complications, including PID. The association between BV and PID is interesting but whether the increasing awareness and management of BV may reflect on the overall incidence of PID is yet to be determined.

Prostatitis

Prostatitis refers to a ubiquitous group of disorders that could be better described under the category of:

- Bacterial Prostatitis: Acute Bacterial Prostatitis
  Chronic Bacterial Prostatitis
- Chronic Pelvic Pain Syndrome (Inflamatory); previously called Chronic Non-bacterial Prostatitis
- Chronic Pelvic Pain Syndrome (Non-inflammatory); previously called Prostadodynia.

Acute Bacterial Prostatitis (APP)

Bacterial Prostatitis (Acute or Chronic) is usually caused by typical urinary pathogens (e.g., Klebsiella, Proteus, Escherichia coli) and possibly Chlamydia. The route of their entry to the prostate is unknown but possibly through pelvic lymphatic spread.

The patient presents with systemic symptoms (pyrexia, rigors, malaise, myalgia and/or arthralgia).Severe APP condition progresses to generalised sepsis, with tachycardia, tachypnoea and hypotension. The first presenting symptoms could be confused with urinary tract infections (namely dysuria, frequency and urgency). The symptoms of prostatitis may or may not be prominent. Typically, the patient complains of perineal pain, that may be perceived by the patient at the tip of the penis, lower back or testicles, and/or rectal pain. The prostate is exquisitely tender, focally or diffusely swollen, warm to touch, boggy and/or indurated.

Chronic Bacterial Prostatitis (CBP)

The symptoms and signs of CBP resemble those of Acute Prostatitis but milder. It is the result of recurrent episodes of infection, with or without resolution in-between. The condition of CBP is identified by the recurrent recovery of pathogenic bacteria from prostatic fluid in the absence of urinary tract infection. The organisms are the same as ABP. Staphylococcus aureus, Streptococcus faecalis and/or Enterococci are encountered. Chronic infections could be associated by bacteria that were sequestered in the prostatic tissue, and therefore not amenable to eradication by antibiotics (e.g., Pseudomonas species, Enterococci, Staphylococcus aureus and rarely Anaerobes).

Chronic Pelvic Pain Syndrome (CPPS)

The CPPS typically presents with pain as the predominant complaint (e.g., pelvic, perineal, lower abdominal, rectal, lower back, retro-pubic, testicular and/or penile tip pain); including ejaculatory pain. Discomfort could be significant to the point of interfering with the quality of life. The patient complains of urinary and/or obstructive micturition symptoms (e.g., frequency, urgency, nocturia, incomplete emptying of bladder and/or abnormal flow). There are no systemic symptoms, but significant psychological morbidity. On examination, the prostate is tender but not swollen or boggy.

Inflammatory CPPS is identified by the finding of leukocytes, but no significant number of bacteria, in the prostatic fluid.

Non inflammatory CPPS, have a similar clinical picture, but neither bacteria nor leukocytes are present in the prostatic fluid.

Asymptomatic Inflammatory Prostatitis is the condition of a patient with no prostatic symptoms; with the finding of leukocytes in prostatic fluid during the course of investigations. The condition should be suspected clinically and requires careful evaluation, to exclude urethritis, peri-rectal abscess and/or urinary tract infections.

The underlying aetiology of CPPS may not be defined in retrospect. It is possible that there is more than one aetiological factor, each leading to similar group of symptoms and signs in what we recognise as CPPS. In some patients, there is evidence of urinary outlet obstructions and/or sympathetic nervous system dysfunctions. Urinary outlet obstruction is dentified on urodynamic and cystoscopy. There are patients with concurrent interstitial cystitis. In others, foreign prostatic antigen is identified and an antigen-antibody reaction is postulated. Pelvic floor muscle dysfunction had been demonstrated in some patients. These findings could be consequences rather than causes of CPPS. There is a recognised therapeutic response to antibiotics; but the anti-inflammatory nature of some of these preparations may have an effect of its own.

Investigations

The process of investigations would be guided by the patient's presentation and/or general condition. In Acute Bacterial Prostatitis, a mid-stream urinalysis is usually positive. Prostatic massage is considered a necessary step in making the diagnosis, in selected cases. The idea of massage of an exquisitely tender prostate will not be acceptable to many patients. The clinician should consider the possibility of provoking bacteraemia. The practical value is questionable, since the same pathogens are usually isolated from urine. The three urine samples test (first-void, mid-stream and post-prostatic massage samples) are collected and assessed for microscopy, cultures and antibiotic susceptibility tests. The expressed prostatic secretions could are collected during urethro-cystoscopy.

Findings suggestive of Prostatitis include:
1. Polymorph nuclear cells (PMNL) /High Power Field (HPF) on microscopic examination of Expressed Prostatic Secretions (EPS) or post-massage urine sample.
   PMNL/HPF Ten times or more, than first-void and mid-stream samples is significant
2. Colony count in EPS and post-massage urine sample.
   cColonies of more than ten times that of first-void and mid-stream urine samples is significant.

Urinary tract colonization should be excluded, prior to performing the prostatic massage. Post-micturition residual urinary collection in the bladder, could be excluded by introducing a course of antimicrobial that does not penetrate the prostatic tissue.

Clinical Practicalities

1. Patients with generalised toxic conditions should have samples for blood culture prior to the initiation of antibiotic therapy; to exclude septicaemia and identify antibiotic susceptibility of any cultured organisms, which can guide the review of therapy later.
2. Prostatic massage is valuable in afebrile patients and urine samples before and after massage assist the diagnosis.
3. Trans-rectal Ultrasonography is required, to determine the extent of inflammation (e.g., Seminal Vesiculitis), and/or exclude prostatic or para-rectal abscesses.
4. Cystoscopy may be required to exclude other pathology and could be useful in obtaining trans-urethral samples after prostatic massage, for microbiological investigations.

Treatment of Acute Bacterial Prostatitis (ABP)

The severity and seriousness of ABP requires immediate medical attention and initiation of empirical antibiotic treatment, which may require hospitalisation and parenteral therapy in severe or non-responsive cases. The clinician needs a low threshold for clinical diagnosis and initiation of prompt antibiotic therapy, to avoid progression to Chronic Bacterial Prostatitis. Samples for microbiological investigations prior to therapy are helpful in guiding treatment review, following the antibioticsusceptibility test results. Older patients may suffer urinary retention and a supra-pubic catheter is preferable to a trans-urethral route, to avoid prostatic/urethral damage, bacteraemia and/or septicaemia. In the non-toxic patients, home treatment with oral antibiotic therapy, bed rest, analgesia, hydration and stool softeners is possible.

Fluoroquinolone initial therapy is usually effective and treatment should be continued for some 28 days; if the clinical response is satisfactory. First line alterantives are: Ofloxacin (200 mg twice daily) Ciprofloxacin (500 mg twice daily) or Norfloxacin (400mg twice daily); all for 28 days. Patients who are allergic to Quinolones could be prescribed Doxycycline (100 mg twice daily), Co-trimoxazole (960 mg twice daily) or Trimethoprim (200 mg twice daily); all for 28 days. The patient would benefit from Non-Steroidal Anti-inflammatory drugs, muscle relaxants (e.g., Cyclobenzapine), Alpha-adrenergic blockers and other symptomatic measures (sitz-bath).

In toxic patients, parenteral therapy should be considered, with broad spectrum antibiotics that would affect the likely organisms (e.g., Ampicillin plus Gentamicin); and should continue until the patient is afebrile for 24-48 hours. The results of the bacterial culture and antibiotic susceptibility test should guide further treatment choice. The intravenous antibiotics are followed by oral therapy of Cephalosporins plus Gentamicin, for 4-6 weeks. The success rate of treatment for those with equivocal or negative cultures is low.

Treatment of Chronic Bacterial Prostatitis (CBP)

The choices include Ciprofloxacin (500 mg, orally, twice daily) or, Ofloxacin (200 mg, orally, twice daily) or, Doxycycline (100 mg, orally, twice daily) or, Trimethoprim (200 mg, orally, twice daily), all for 28 days. There is no evidence that treatment for a longer period with antibiotics provides more benefit.

Clinical Practicalities

1. The diagnosis of Prostatitis is based mainly on symptoms; as signs could be inconclusive.
2. Patients with acute bacterial prostatitis require investigations, after the acute episode, to exclude underlying abnormalities of the urinary tract. The patient would benefit from urinary tract ultrasonography and possibly intravenous –urogram.
3. Patients with ABP who are treated in out-patient require assessment three days after initiation of treatment to review clinical improvement The patient may need hospitalisation and intravenous antibiotics, if there is deterioration in the clinical condition.
4. Occult prostatic infection is difficult to exclude. Antibiotic treatment may prove effective due to the anti-inflammatory effect of some drugs (e.g., Tetracyclines).
5. The non-steroidal anti-inflammatory agents have therapeutic benefits, in addition to their symptomatic relief.
6. Lack of response to adequate treatment should raise the suspicion of the possibility of prostatic abscess which may require aspiration, evacuation and drainage.

7. Many Prostatic Abscesses are discovered incidentally, during prostatic surgery or endoscopy; including rupture during instrumentation.
8. Selective Alpha-blockers could be valuable, if there is evidence of urinary outlet obstruction. The clinical response provides guidance to their continued and long-term use.

The Management of Patients with Chronic Pelvic Pain Syndrome (CPPS) [Inflamatory & Non-Inflamatory]

The diagnosis of CPPS is made retrospectively, following a history of recurrent episodes. Asking the patient to keep Pain Diary will help the diagnosis, provide a measure of the patient's frequency, severity and duration of symptoms and response to treatment. The patient would usually have had investigations and treatment for prostatitis, including three urine samples tests, pelvic/trans-rectal ultra-sonography, urethro-cystoscopy, prostatic massage, uro-dynamic studies and/or repeated courses of antibiotics.

The treatment modalities are still under scrutiny. There are reports of benefits, but the patient should be warned of the chronic nature of CPPS and its long term care plane. The following therapeutic options prove valuable: Muscle Relaxants, to counter-act pelvic floor dysfunction, Selective Serotonin Re-uptake Inhibitors (SSRIs), to modulate the perception of pain, pelvic microwave/heat therapy, to induce hyperaemia, Benzodiazepines, to counteract anxiety and/or sacral nerve stimulation, to reverse referred pain. Different combinations of therapy were reported to be beneficial, for selected patients.

Epididymo-Orchitis

Epididymitis may be localised, generalised or accompanied by inflammation of the testicles (epididymo-orchitis). The offending organism may gain access to the bladder and/or urethra, by trans-cavity spread through the ejaculatory duct, seminal vesicle and vas-deference, or through lymphatics or blood vessels; from distant origins. In the sexually active, under 35 years of age, C trachomatis and N gonorrhoea are the leading cause. It is estimated that 1 in 3 patients with untreated urethritis may progress to epididymitis. In Western countries and where sexual health services are available, the early diagnosis and treatment of STIs expectedly lead to decline in associated epididymo-orchitis. In men aged over 35, Coliform bacteria (i.e., Escherichia coli, Klepsidilla and Proteus species) are leading causes. It may be associated with urinary tract infections and/or underlying urological abnormalities (e.g., obstructions or calculus), indwelling catheters or recent urological procedures. Tuberculous Epididymitis, Syphilitic Gummas and Mycotic Epididymitis (i.e., Actinomycosis, Plastomycosis) are becoming scarce with the improved diagnosis and treatment of thier systemic conditions. They may still be encountered in immuno-compromised patient (HIV). Retrograde flow of urine into the epididymis, during Valsalva's manoeuvre (e.g., digging and heavy lifting) may lead to chemical/non-bacterial epididymitis.

The diagnosis is based on clinical assessment. Scrotal pain is a predominant symptom, irrespective of the aetiology being bacterial or non-bacterial. Severe scrotal pain may radiate to the abdomen or inner side of the thigh. There may be associated fever, nausea and/or urinary symptoms in bacterial Epididymitis; or urethral discharge, dysuria and frequency, if associated with Urethritis. Clinical examination reveals swelling and tenderness of the epididymis and adjacent testicle. There may be signs and laboratory indicators of urethritis or urinary tract infection.

Practical Considerations

1. Presentation of Testicular Torsion may mimic epididymo-orchitis and the condition should be proactively considered and excluded due to the serious consequences of delayed intervention. The prior history of sudden movement, the acute occurrence and ultrasonographic/doplar findings, direct the diagnosis of testicular torsion. The affected testicle is tender and may be elevated in a horizontal position, with absence of the cremasteric reflex on the affected side. Manual correction (de-torsion) is successful in some 30-70% of cases. The procedure of de-torsion could be guided by extent of pain.The correction is performed in an outward direction and more than one rotation may be needed. If unsuccessful, the patient should have immediate surgery for correction and fixation.
    Fixation of both testicles is usually required, as the anatomical defect is bilateral.
2. The clinician should not presume the cause of epididymo-orchitis is sexually transmitted; although STIs needs to be proactively considered and excluded by investigations.
3. Inflammation may be part of the generalised condition (e.g., Behcet's Disease) or a side-effect to drugs (e.g., Amiodarone).
4. Leakage of spermatozoa into testicular tissue (e.g., following trauma) may lead to auto-immune reaction, inflammation, granulomatous changes and fibrosis.
5. Chronic epididymo-orchitis with granulomatous changes may be part of a generalised disorder (e.g., idiopathic or associated with sarcoidosis).
6. Mumps induced orchitis is estimated to affect 1 in 5 post-pubertal males affected with mumps. The inflammation is usually unilateral and may lead to some testicular atrophy. Testosterone production and fertility are usually preserved, contrary to public beliefs.
7. Epididymitis and/or Orchitis may be part of allergic lymphangitis and oedema following filariasis and elephantiasis.
8. Males practising insertive anal sex who have non-gonococcal, non-chlamydial epididymitis have a chance of coliform enteric bacteria as the underlying cause.

The Herpes Simplex Virus and Herpes Genitalis

The Virus

The Herpes Simplex Virus (HSV) is a neurotropic virus with predilection to muco-cutaneous junctions. Type 1 (HSV-1) affects the Oro-labial mucosa and Type 2 (HSV-2) has a predilection mainly to the genital mucosa. There appears to be an increasing number of genital lesions encountered in clinical practice that are biologically attributed to HSV-1; most likely due to increasing practice of oral sex. The prevalence of either types relate to socio-economic status, age, onset of coitarch and/or practice of oral sex. The prevalence of the virus in a given community could be as high as 80%.

The estimated HSV-2 infections in the USA are in the region of 50 millions; with some 700,000 new clinical cases/ year. One in three of the 30-40 years old is estimated to be infected with HSV-2.

The rate of diagnosed first attack of genital herpes, in the UK, varied with sex and county. The average was 36/100,00 population in 2006. The HPA recorded some 21,000 new diagnosis of genital Herpes, in UK GUM clinics, for year 2006 (31% increase from 1997). Rates were higher in women. The highest rates were in the 20-24 years age group, for both men and women (108 and 223/100,000 population, respectivly). Regional variations were stark. The highest rates were for London and Metropolitan cities.

There are studies for HSV-2 prevelance in other developing communities; with reported rates varying from 2-80%; depending on age, sex, urbanization and sexual practices.

The Virus

HSV is a relatively large virus, measuring 200nm. It has an envelop of lipid and glycoprotein, an intermediate layer of viral proteins and an icosahedral capsid, containing the double stranded DNA genome.

Transmission

The virus is vulnerable to desiccation and temperature and therefore requires direct intimate contact. Transmission by fomites and fluids is theoretically possible but very unlikely. The virus requires a breach in the mucocutaneous surfaces, as small as a microscopic one. The neurotropic nature of the virus leads to a period of dormancy; where the virus resides in the dorsal root ganglia of the sensory nerves of the affected dermatome.

Clinical Presentation

Reactivation of the virus, provoked by stress, fever, immuno-suppression, menstruation, trauma and/or ultra-violet light, leads to a lesion. The lesion may be detectable by the patient (symptomatic) and the clinician (clinical lesion). Otherwise, the condition may not be detectable by the patient (asymptomatic) or the clinician (sub-clinical lesion). Reactivation is associated with viral shedding. This explain how a patient may acquire infection from a partner who may not be aware of his/her positive herpes status (i.e in asymptomatic shedding). The majority of infections are acquired from patients who are infected, but not symptomatic. Similarly, the majority of new patients who acquire the infection are asymptomatic.

The incubation period ranges from 1-40 days. Some patients may develop generalised symptoms (e.g., raised temperature, photophobia, headache and/or malaise); which occurs usually in primary episodes. Some patients give history of topical prodromal symptoms (e.g., tingling) at the site of the lesion, prior to the appearance of the vesicles. The vesicles progress to pustules, then to superficial multiple ulcers, surrounded with erythema and/or oedema. The lesion persists for few days, but may persist for up to two weeks. Without viral suppression, additional crops of successive lesions may reappear within the first week. The lesion may take three weeks to resolve. If complicated with secondary infection, the lesions may continue for weeks.

Past exposure to HSV infection leads to immunological memory, which reduces the severity of symptoms of subsequent secondary episodes. A prodromal stage is recognised by some patients (e.g., pain, feeling of pins, needles and tingling), inguinal pain and/or sciatic neuralgia. The severity of lesions vary; but in some unfortunate cases could be extensive enough to cause psychological implications, which add to the patient's generalised distress and perpetuate a cycle of vulnerability. There is a theoretical possibility of auto-inoculation, possibly leading to eye infection and kerato-conjunctivitis. Skin breaches can lead to extra genital lesions in the surrounding areas (e.g., groin, buttocks and/or lips); or distant contact (e.g., fingers). The condition may lead to generalised eczematous skin changes. Peri-anal infection may follow anal sex and lead to herptic lesions. The most significant complication is the psychological impact. This was more pronounced when there were inaccurate medical comments of a relationship between genital herpes and cervical cancers. Early reports, in the 70s and 80s, promoted the idea of an association between HSV and cervical cancer. This caused anxiety and could be traced in some patients until now. The clinician should encourage patients to reach for up-to-date knowledge, to expel the myth and unfounded anxiety.

Complications with secondary bacterial infections can take place and should be avoided with attention to hygiene; otherwise be actively treated. Urinary retention may be the result of severe pain and/or neuropathy. Immuno-compromised patients carry the risk of HSV disseminated infections. Meningeal irritation, associated with HSV infection, suggests viral spread by viraemia. Ulcers on two opposing surfaces (e.g sub-preputial and glans or two sides of vulval labiae [kissing ulcers]) can coalesce and lead to amalgamations and adhesions.

Genital herpes is one of the commonest genital ulcerative diseases and a major cofactor in HIV infection. Genital ulcerations are significant co-factor in HIV spread and acquisition of new infection. A breach in the skin or mucus surface promotes the HIV virus access to the recipient's human body.

Recurrences are common with HSV-2; where most patients have 3-4 recurrences per year; and may extend for years in some patients. In HSV-1infections, half of the patients have 2 recurrences per year. Ano-genital herpes caused by HSV-1 is less likely to recur and is confined to the first year in most occurrences. The area affected is usually the same site of the previous primary attack; but smaller with a shorter clinical course. The severity of the primary attack is suggestive of the future frequency, recurrences and their intensity. Immuno-compromised patients are vulnerable to recurrences and severe episodes.

Early childhood herpes genitalis should pose the question of the possibility of child sexual abuse. Transmission through fomites and inanimate objects is possible but not likely. The virus inactivate readily in room temperature and drying. Therefore close contact with a fresh and large inocculum is essential for transmission to take place. For the same reasons, auto-inoculation is possible but not common. Direct contact is the most likely route of transmission; therefore the possibility of sexual contact should be considered.

Diagnosis

Tests to confirm the diagnosis of herpes genitalis require time; and the patient's distress requires the early initiation of treatment. An experienced clinician would make a provisional clinical diagnosis and initiate empirical treatment, prior to virological confirmation. The clinician must explain to the patient that virological confirmation is necessary, to make a confirmed diagnosis. Awaiting results can delay what could be a window of therapeutic opportunity.

Viral culture has a high sensitivity but requires vesicular fluid. They are not suitable for lesions with scabs and may report false negative if the patient has applied antiseptic material to the lesion. Some Viral Transport Media may require refrigeration. It is prudent to follow the manufacturer's instructions and keep communications with the local microbiology laboratory.

Immuno-Fluorescent (IF) tests for viral antigen, have lower sensitivity but provide a quick result that could be of value in some clinical situations (e.g., during delivery and the early neo-natal period).

The finding of multi-nucleic giant cells, on cytology smears of lesional samples, is of theoretical interest but little practical application; due to its demand on staff and time resources.

Polymerase Chain Reaction (PCR) tests provide the most sensitive method and can identify positive cases in over 80% of cases, at an early stage. The test is rapid, but there are cost implications, which could be reduced by multiple testing in centralised laboratories.

Type specific Herpes simplex virus serology has defined but restricted clinical value and requires carefull clinical interpretation.

The Complement Fixation Test (CFT) and identification of IgM antibody could help the diagnosis in late presentation; when Lesional swabs are not likely to be productive. Ig M is valuable for the diagnosis of Herpes neo-natorum.

Treatment

The management depends on early clinical diagnosis and informed discussion between the patient and the clinician, regarding the options. Emotional support is important and the provision of information, verbal, leaflets and web resources, could allay myths, fears and anxieties. The HSV "Patient Support Group" provide information and emotional assistance.

Systemic antiviral treatment has the benefit of reducing intensity of attacks, period of symptoms and viral shredding. It should start as early as possible, as the benefits are less for healing lesions. The options are: Aciclovir (200 mg, orally, five times daily or 400 mg twice daily), Famciclovir (250 mg, orally, three times daily) or Valaciclovir (500 mg, orally,. twice daily), all for five days.

A severe and extensive primary lesion would require a higher dosage and longer period of treatment. A severe disease (e.g., disseminated infection with pneumonitis, hepatitis, meningitis and/or encephalitis) necessitates hospitalisation and intravenous therapy in the form of Acyclovir (5-10mg/kg body weight, IV, every eight hours) until clinical improvement (usually 2-7 days). This should be followed by oral therapy to complete at least ten days course. Allergic and adverse reactions to therapy are rare and would require desensitisation to Acyclovir.

Suppressive herpes antiviral therapy has a place for patients with recurrent episodes leading to distress. There is value in therapeutic respite, when a patient may require the treatment to avoid episodes during special occasions (e.g., a Honeymoon or a holiday). There is also a value for a respite, to break the cycle of recurrent episodes. Frequent recurrences lead to distress and increase the patient's vulnerability to HSV; with the possibility of more episodes. There is an alternative option of episodic treatment, where the patient may carry a supply to use at the earliest onset of symptoms. It has a place in less recurrent episodes (e.g., six episodes/ year). Episodic therapy carries a risk of over use. As a result of patient's distress, symptoms resulting from another condition can lead to apprehension and misinterpretation as a herpetic attack. A clinical and virological confirmation of recurrences should be achieved, prior to commitment to suppressive therapy. The access and availability of local services, for clinical confirmation and early treatment, balances the options of therapeutic regimens. The distress associated with six confirmed recurrences of herpes genitalis, in a year, is an indication of suppressive treatment. There needs to be an agreement between the patient and the clinician regarding the duration of treatment, as there is a possibility of recurrences after cessation of therapy. What neither the patient nor the clinician would like to reach is a state of continuous dependence and intake of suppressive therapy. There are benefits in discussing general health measures, for reducing the level of stress and avoide HSV predisposing factors. The suppressive therapy regimen includes Aciclovir (400mg, orally, twice daily), Famciclovir (250mg, orally, twice daily), and Valaciclovir (500mg, orally, once daily), for a period of three to six months.

Herpes Simplex and Pregnancy

Primary HSV attack during pregnancy caries high risk of foetal transmission and infection; in the absence of protective effect of maternal herpes specific antibodies. The effect may range from foetal demise to variable degrees of Herpes Neonatorum. The effects may be less significant if the infection takes place at a stage when antibodies had an opportunity to develp (i.e., over three months). Primary attacks closer to delivery are serious; and active genital tract lesions during delivery cary the highest risk of transmission. Most obstetricians and mothers would elect for caesarean section delivery; to avoid foetal exposure to active genital tract HSV lesions. Ther is evidence to suggest that rupture of foetal membranes of four hours or more increases the chances of transmission. Herpes Neonatorum is managed with intravenous Aciclovir.

Neo-natal herpes is a serious condition and is registrable in the UK. The incidence is 1.6/100,000 live births in the UK; compared with 11.4/100,000 in California, USA. The highest risk is a maternal primary attack close to the time of delivery. It is presumed that mothers with recurrent / secondary attacks, develop and transfer a degree of immunity to the foetus/newborn. The reduced shedding and frequency of attacks, following past maternal exposure, could be a contributing factor. There had been a practice of clinical examinations and inspecting the cervix in the later weeks of pregnancy, to identify lesions that could be due to herpes genitalis.The practice proved unhelpeful, as it does not exclude sub-clinical lesions and/or asymptomatic shedding. There was also a practice of taking cervical swabs for HSV virology tests; on weekly basis. HSV swabs proved to be of little clinical or practical value, due to the time lag between the obstetric event and obtaining the virology results.

There could be a place for suppressive therapy in the last trimester of pregnancy, which could reduce recurrences and shedding. Aciclovir is not licensed for use in pregnancy but there is a body of clinical experience for its antenatal intake. Aciclovir (200 mg orally four times daily; or 400 mg three times daily), is given during the last four weeks of pregnancy. The pros and cons of the different options benefit from an informed discussion between the patient, obstetrician and STI clinician.

Secondery attacks, theoretically, are less serious. The HSV specific antibodies should give a degree of protection and immunity to the foetus and newborn. The risk is very small. The decision of management should be the result of informed discussions between the mother and clinicians. Caesarean section transfers risk from the foetus to the mother; and some patients elect to take four weeks of suppressive therapy.

The Clinical Value of Serology Tests for Herpes Simplex

Type specific serological tests for Herpes, for HSV-1 or HSV-2 confer clinical values in the following situation:

1)   A patient who has history of clinical lesions, that proved to be due to HSV, should be advised to inform his/her sex partner. The non-symptomatic partner may wish to identify his/her HSV status and whether s/he had a previous infection leading to sub-clinical and/or asymptomatic episodes. Serology tests could define the HSV concordance, or otherwise, in a partnership.

2)   A pregnant woman, with no history of previous herpetic genital ulcerations, and a discordant sex partner (i.e., a partner with a history of oral/labial and/or genital lesions, that proved to be due to HSV) would benefit from identifying her HSV serological status. HSV serology tests would identify whether she had been infected with HSV (e.g., asymptomatic or sub-clinical lesions). Past exposure to HSV and harbouring HSV type specific antibodies, will confer a degree of protection and immunity to the mother and the newborn. If she is otherwise expressing negative HSV serology tests, which suggest no past exposure, she would be at risk of primary herpetic

attack during pregnancy; which puts the newborn at a higher risk of Herpes Neonatorum. The couple in this case would have the opportunity of making an informed choice on the sexual practices they may, or may not wish to have, to avoid HSV transmission and the possibility of a primary attack during pregnancy.The couple may wish to abstain from sexual intercourse during pregnancy and would benefit from an informed choice.

3)   A pregnant woman who who had a history of genital lesions, that are similar to herpes genitalis; but had no past history of confirmation of HSV, could benefit from serology tests. There is a possibility that she has had past asymptomatic/sub-clinical lesions and therefore her episodes are going to be secondary; that were made prominent due to pregnancy. HSV serology will indicate past exposure and therefore help the diagnosis of a secondary attack; indicate that she harbours HSV specific antibodies; and therefore transefer immunity and confer protection to the newborn. Ther could be a very small risk to the neonate from maternal secondary herpetic episodes that take place during delivery.

4)   A patient who has recurrent genital ulcerations that are clinically suspicious of herpes; but has repeated negative culture or PCR tests for HSV. Lesional swabs, for HSV viral culture may erroneously and repeatedly report negative (i.e., false negative). The introduction of PCR for HSV lesional tests, where available, could to confirm the diagnosis of HSV. A positive HSV serology could help the differential diagnosis. A positive test would support the diagnosis of Herpes Genitalis. A negative serology excludes HSV and diverts attention to other clinical conditions (e.g., Genital Aphthous Ulcerations). Recurrent genital ulcerations may present with lesions resembling HSV type ulcers; but caused by another aetilogy. The treatment for Genital Aphthous Ulcers is based on strong topical steroids. Given erroneously in a case of HSV ulcers, topical steroids may worsen the clinical condition. Recurrent genital ulcerations with negative HSV serology tests, is not likely to be caused by HSV.

The above mentioned clinical situations are very complex and require high degree of clinical, virological and serological skills, and expertise, to reach an accurate assessment and conclusion. The identification of IgG and IgM can differentiate a past from a recent infection.

Bacterial Vaginosis

Bacterial vaginosis (BV) is not an infection, but an overgrowth of vaginal commensal bacteria (Gardenerella vaginalis, Anaerobic bacteria and Microplasmas); with a shift of balance from the Lactobacillus species. Gardener and Duke described the condition as "non-specific Vaginitis", in 1955, hence the name of Gardenerella vaginalis. The condition was later known as Bacterial Vaginosis (BV), to confirm that vaginal inflammation is not a pathological entity of the condition. The hydrogen peroxide producing lactobacilli confer protection from BV and women having these organisms are less effected by BV, han their counterparts.

The presence of BV is higher in non-caucasians, sexually active, smokers, those who practise vaginal douching or use intrauterine device (IUD). One in ten virgins may also suffer BV. G vaginalis is commonly found in the urethras of male partners of females affected with BV. There is no need to provide concurrent treatment to the male, as it does not reduce recurrences in a female partner with BV. The relationship between BV and sexual intercourse is one of association rather than causation. It is possible that the alkaline nature of semen interferes with the vaginal acidity and predisposes to conditions favouring BV. This is also supported by the observation that BV is commoner in lesbians practising receptive genital oral sex (cunnilingus) The alkalinity of the salivary fluid could disrupt normal vaginal acidity and leading to in changes in vaginal floral balance.

The growth of organisms, in patients with BV, increases to more than 100 times the normal concentration. The prevailing organisms are anaerobic, facultative, Gram negative bacilli. They could also be isolated in two thirds of females with normal discharge. The Mobiluncus species, which is anaerobic, sickle shaped rods), are found in up to 95% of women with BV. Mycoplasma hominis is found in up to three quarters females with BV, but are also present in patients without BV. Other organisms implicated in BV include Bacteroids, Pepto-streptococci, Fusobacterium and Prevotella species. Atopobium vaginae is newly-identified Metronidazole resistance Gram positive anaerobe; and may explain treatment failures in some patients. Aerobic bacteria (α and β Haemolytic Streptococci and Coliforms) are also implicates in cases of BV.

Clinical Presentation

BV is a very common cause for vaginal discharge with prevalence ranging from 5 to 50%, according to the study population. The patient usually presents with vaginal discharge; that is described as homogenous, grey to white, moderate in amount and frothy. The patient and/or her partner may report a fishy smell following sexual intercourse and ejaculation. She may experience the problem during menstruation, due to increased vaginal ph with alkaline menstrual fluids. BV could be associated with N gonorrhoea, C trachomatis, NSU and/or Trichomoniasis.

BV is associated with pelvic inflammatory disease, occurring spontaneously or following a procedure (e.g., insertion of intra-uterine contraceptive device or abortion). It can lead to infections following pelvic surgery. During pregnancy, the production of cytokines and prostaglandins by the incumbent bacteria is associated with chorioamnionitis, low birth weight, pre-term delivery, premature rupture of membranes, and/or post-partum endometritis.

Diagnosis

The presence of three or more of the following (Amsel Criteria) fulfils the diagnosis of BV: characteristic discharge, the release of fishy smelling amines on mixing 10% Potassium Hydroxide with a sample of vaginal fluid on a glass slide, vaginal pH higher than 4.5 and/or the presence of vaginal clue cells on Gram stained vaginal smear. The Gram staining and microscopic reading of vaginal smear is simple and accurate bed side test. The typical appearance is Gram variable bacilli adhering to vaginal epithelial cells, which is knowb as "Clue Cells". The slide will show other Gram negative Bacilli and Gram positive Cocci; with a clear reduction of Lactobacilli.

Nugent Criteria is the quantitative scoring for Lactobacilli, G vaginalis, Bacteroids and/or Mobiluncus on a microscopy read, Gram-stained, vaginal smear. A score of 6 or above identifies BV. A score of 3 or below identifies normal vaginal conditions; and a score between 4 and 6 is intermediate.

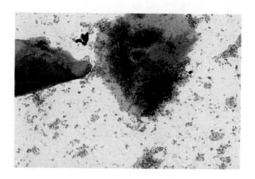

Figure 1. Gram-stained Microscopy slide showing Clue cells

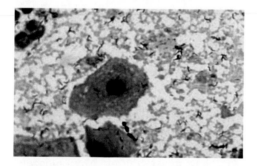

Figure 2. Gram-stained Microscopy slide showing Vaginal Epithelial cells

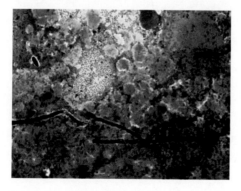

Figure 3. Gram-stained Microscopy slide showing Hyphae and Clue cells

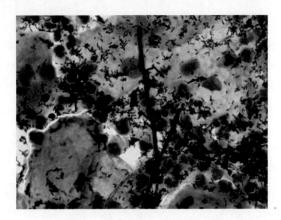

Figure 4. Gram-stained Microscopy slide showing Hyphae

Management

Fifty percent of the patients suffering with BV are asymptomatic and for whom treatment is questionable. For symptomatic patients, their cure rate is high with Metronidazole (400 mg, orally, twice daily for 7 days or 2 g as a single dose) or Metronidazole vaginal gel (0.75%, 5 gm/applicator, per vaginum, once daily, for 5 days). Alternatively, Clindamycin (300 mg, orally, twice daily, for 7 days) or Clindamycin vaginal cream (2%, one applicator daily for 7 days) or Clindamycin vaginal pessary (100 mg, daily for 3 days) or Tinidazole (2g, oral, in a single dose) could be used. Clindamycin may weaken condoms and the patient should be warned. Alcohol intake during Metronidazole treatment lead to disulfiram like effect and should be avoided

Practical Issues for Recurrent/Persistent BV

1. The effect of alkaline fluids (e.g., semen, saliva, bath water/soap) on the vaginal pH, and its possible distortion of the vaginal acidity should be explained to the patient. Simple changes in habits can lead to appreciable improvement.
2. There is no medical indication to treat the male partner of a patient diagnosed with BV.
3. There could be benefits of investigating the condition of the female partner in a gay relationship due to the higher possibility of BV with

insertive vaginal-oral sex. The couple may wish to reconsider insertive vaginal-oral sex as a way of reducing BV recurrences.

4. Contraceptive methods that reduce menstrual flow (e.g Progesterone only contraception) could avoid higher ph associated with menstruation.

5. Alternative therapy should be considered (e.g., change from Metronidazole to Clindamycin and vise versa).

6. Co-amoxiclav [Amoxicillin 250mg plus Clavulanic Acid 125mg] (orally, three times daily for seven days), could be used; to counter-act the possible deactivation of Mitronidazole by other bacteria implicated with persitant BV.

Bacterial vaginosis during Pregnancy

There is an association between BV and early pregnancy loss, chorio-amnionitis, premature rupture of membranes, pre-term delivery and small for date foetus. The early diagnosis and treatment of BV during pregnancy is indicated; but routine screening for asymptomatic pregnanat women is not justified. During pregnancy, treatment with Clindamycin is of particular interest; due to precautions with Metronidazole use.

Vulvo-Vaginal Candidiasis (VVC)

The Causative Organism/s

Vulvo-Vaginal Candidiasis (VVC), commonly known as thrush or moniliasis, is caused by the activity of commensal Fungi. It affect patients with reduced systemic and/or local immunity, but more often affect patients with no underlying clear cause. Candida albicans is the causative agent in some 90% of cases. Candida glabrata is the cause in another 5-10%; with other fungi rarely attributed to the condition. The organism multiplies by budding from fungus cells (Blastospores, approx 1-5 μm). C albicans produce multiple cell units (hyphae), in the form of tubes divided by septa and rise from the fungus cell or branches (i.e., from another existing hyphae). C albicans may have single elongated cell, budding from the yeast cell and remaining attached to it (pseudo-hyphae). C albicans may have large bodies with double cell wall and is thought to be a dormant phase (Chlamydospores).

C glabrata have no hyphae or pseudo-hyphae. The pathogenic nature of the organism is enhanced by its ability of mucosal adherence, by its surface molecules, mucous disintegration, by proteases and invasion of the mucosal wall by hyphae and germ tubes. The ability of the organism to function as commensal, its ability to develop spores and dormant phases and/or its production of penetrative hyphae and germ tubes, all contribute into recurrences.

Transmission

The commensal nature of the Candida species account for its recovery from the mouth, vagina and/or ano-rectal cannel in a third of individuals; which contribute to recurrences and lack of permanent cures. The rule of coitus as a factor in transmission and precipitation of vulvo-vaginal candidiasis is notable but unclear. Theoretically, peno-vaginal intercourse may transmit the organisms from the peri-anal area into the vagina, precipitate mucosal damage and/or change the vaginal pH from acidic into alkaline (by the alkalinity of semen). The cumulative effect is the precipitation and promotion of vulvo-vaginal candidiasis. It remains unclear why some patients are more vulnerable than others, whilst the above factors could be common to both groups of individuals. The effect of oro-vaginal sex may also be co-factor in vulvo-vaginal candidiasis; by effect of transmission of the oral fungi, moistering the vulval or vaginal mucosa and/or interfering with vaginal acidity by the alkaline saliva). There is evidence of cross-association of VVC and other STIs and non-specific genital infections. A third of male partners of female patients affected by VVC, present with Balano-Posthitis. The management of mild Candidal Balano-Posthitis could simply by achieved by genital hygiene, saline irrigation and barrier contraception (condoms).

Predisposing and Precipitating Factors

The understanding factors that predispose VVC help to avoide and/or reduce recurrences. Impaired immunity (e.g., HIV, chemotherapy or corticosteroid therapy) are predisposing factor; but accounts for a small percentage of patients presenting in clinical settings. A small group of patients report VVC, following the intake of broad spectrum antibiotics; but the majority of those taking the drugs do not report symptoms of VVC. Uncontrolled Diabetes Mellitus, by virtue of supplying the organism with glucose, for its energy consumption, precipitates VVC and recurrences. VVC is notable more in females within the child-bearing period. VVC is less common in pre-menarcheal girls and post-menopausal women. The higher oestrogen levels increase the vaginal glycogen content and provide a milieu conducive for yeast growth. Patients using the high dose oestrogen contraceptive pill report more episodes of VVC. VVC could be encountered in female neonates, secondary to the effect of maternal oestrogen. It affect post-menopausal woman who are using oestrogen for Hormone Replacement Therapy. VVC is reported more during the Luteal Phase of the menstrual cycle; with premenstrual flares. The higher progesterone level during the Luteal phase causes relative immuno-suppression. Progesterone and oestrogen surges during pregnancy contribute to the ante-natal vulnerability to VVC and its recurrences. The effect of the spermicidal agents, on lowering the population of Lactobacilli, and contributing to VVC, is controversial. The use of diaphragms and caps carry the possibility of fungal contamination and re-infection. There is no clear proof that the use of condoms can prevent recurrences, but there are merits of using it to prevent the alteration of the vaginal acidity by the alkaline semen, in patients suffering VVC recurrences. Whether the commulative effect of genital perspiration, containment by tight synthetic underwear, increased genital temperature and subsequent humidity, contribute into VVC recurrences, is unproven. Reversing these conditions in patients who are plagued with VVC recurrences is a measure worth taking, on empirical grounds.

There are association between Chronic Muco-Cutaneous Candidiasis and patients with severe anaemia or auto-immune conditions (e.g., Addison's diseases, Hypo-thyroidism and Hypo-para-thyroidism). The relationship is rare but worth considering clinically.

Clinical Presentation

Women presenting with VVC symptoms complain of vulval soreness, burning, itching, vaginal discharge, Dysuria and/or superficial Dyspareunia. The majority of VVC cases are acute episodes. Some patients give history of a cyclical pattern (e.g., Luteal phase symptoms, worsening in the premenstrual period). The physical signs vary in intensity, ranging from vulval erythema at the muco-cutaneous junction, to severe inflammation extending to the surrounding labia and perineum. Satellite erythematous lesions are pathognomonic of Candidiasis. Skin fissures, appearing like epidermal cracks, are characteristic of VVC; and add to the patient's Dysuria, Dyspareunia and distress. The typical discharge is thick, white and curdy. The discharge is prominent in pregnant women and may form plaques adherent to the vaginal wall. Multiple vaginal infections, can lead to purulent or watery discharge; according to the nature of concurrent infection/s.

Recurrent Vulvo-Vaginal Candidiasis (RVVC) is a challenging diagnosis. The availability of over-the-counter medications gives patients the opportunity of self-diagnosis and treatment of Recurrent VVC; many of whom will not exhibit laboratory evidence of the condition. A proportion of these patients are likely to be suffering from a different cause of vulval burning and/or soreness (e.g., eczema or Lichen Sclerosous), that is misperceived as recurrent VVC. It is important that the diagnosis of RVVC is made on clinical and laboratory assessment, to avoid wrong diagnosis and unnecessary courses of treatment. It is necessary to review the patient's condition, following her recovery from the acute inflammatory stage; to re-assess the underlying vulval skin. There could be an underlying skin disease, that is concealed by the erythema and oedema caused by VVC; and predisposes to its recurrences (e.g., Vulval Lichen Sclerosous).

Recurrent VVC could be the result of inadequate or incomplete treatment and reduced local vulvo- vaginal immunity. The episodes are precipitated by the predisposing factors mentioned above. There is a correlation between RVVC and cyclical allergic conditions (e.g., Allergic Rhinitis), hence hypersensitivity factors are considered. The four fold increased involvement of male partners, of women affected by RVVC, suggest a correlation with sexual intercourse.

Male partners may present with evidence of penile glans inflammation (Balanitis) and/or inflammation of prepuce (Posthitis). Balanitis presents as erythematous rash, occasionally with white papules or plaques. The mild forms exhibit aceto-white plaques, on the application of a cotton soaked with 3-5% acetic acid. The plaques could be confused with, and need to be differentiated from, sub-clinical HPV or intra-epithelial dysplasia.

Chronic Vulvo-Vaginal Candidiasis is common in the obese, diabetics and the elderly. It could be complicated by superimposed acute exacerbations. It leads to vulval skin lichenification and requires a long period of therapy.

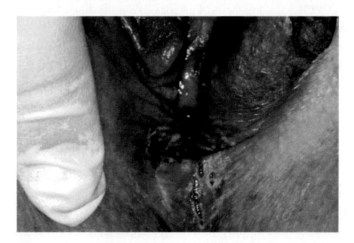

Figure 1. Localized Vulvitis and Skin Cracks

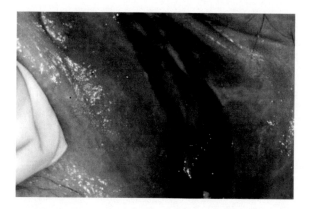

Figure 2. Severe Vulvitis and Oedema

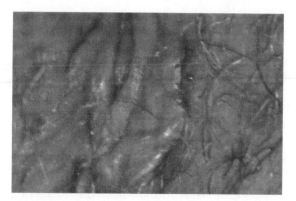

Figure 3. Subacute Vulvitis and Skin Cracks

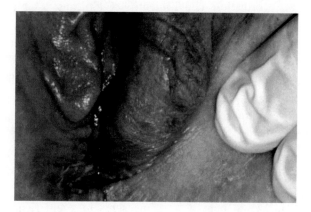

Figure 4. Vulvitis and Left sided Oedema

Diagnosis

Diagnosis relies on the clinical picture, supported by laboratory tests. Self-diagnosis is unreliable; as the patients' distress and anxiety leads to over-diagnosis. The microbiology samples require materials from the discharge and/or inflammatory areas. A moistened cotton tiped swab, or a plastic loop, could be used to obtain samples for microscopy and culture tests. The material could be inoculated directly into the growth medium (e.g., Sabouraud); or sent in a transport medium (e.g., Amies).

Recurrent VVC in HIV Patients

The carriage rate of C albicans in HIV patients increases to almost 90%, in the oro-pharynx or vagina. Recurrent vulvo-vaginal candidiasis in HIV patients is not an indicator on its own and usually responds to conventional treatment. There is a possibility of resistance to Fluconazole, in HIV patients with RVVC, which should be considered in the choice of therapy.

Clinical Practicalities

1. Culture alone is not enough for the diagnosis of VVC, as the yeasts are commencals and colonisation affects up to 20% of the population.
2. Germ tube formation could identify C.albicans; C glabrata do not develop hyphae.
3. Culture can identify the species and consequently guide therapy.
4. Direct Microscopy of saline wet-mounted preparation can identify pseudo-hyphae and/or spores; which could also be identified on Gram-stained smears. C.glabrata produce spores only but no hyphae.
5. Skin scrapings could be used for the preparation of Gram-stained smears, for microscopy, or cultures.
6. The microscopy and culture tests are not done in isolation but as part of a comprehensive investigation of the patient's condition. Concurrent other STIs should be considered and excluded.
7. The patient would benefit from measures to avoid rising genital skin humidity and temperature (e.g., tight, synthetic clothes and underwear).

She should be adviced to avoid conditions that may produce additional hyper-sensitivity (e.g., perfumed products).

8. Saline genital wash/bath has the benefit of discouraging fungal overgrowth, due to high osmolarity and its effect on the organism.

9. The use of vulval skin moisturising agents have a beneficial soothing effect.

10. The patient's choice on the route of drug administration should be considered. There are good clinical responses to either topical and/or oral preparations.

11. Topical creams have a soothing effect.

12. Topical anti-mycotics containing hydrocortisone could be used for short periods. These have the advantage of symptomatic relief when there are hyper sensitivity reactions. They carry the disadvantage of masking underlying pathology (e.g., mild Vulval Lichen Sclerosous), which could be the predisposing factor to RVVC.

13. The suspicion of underlying vulval dermatological conditions (e.g., Lichen Sclerosous) should withhold the use of topical steroids, until a confirmed diagnosis is made. Steroids may distort the clinical and/or histological pictures of the underlying dermatological condition.

14. The possible damage to latex condoms by topical preparations should be explained to the patient.

15. There are Anecdotal reports of benefits from alternative-medicine; but without evidence based conclusions.

16. Drug resistance is common with C glabrata (e.g.,Clotrimazole, Miconazole).

17. Nystatin resistance is rare and there are benefits of its use with C glabrata infection

Treatment of VVC: Anti-Mycotics

External: Clotrimazole cream (1% and 2%, topically, three times daily), or Econazole cream (1%, twice daily) or Ketoconazole cream (2% twice daily) or Miconazole cream (2% twice daily),or Nystatin cream (100,000U/g, four times daily), all for 7-10 days.

Clotrimazole, Econazole and Nystatin are also available in preparations containing Hydrocortisone.

Intra-vaginal preparations could be used in addition to the external creams as there is concurrent Candidal Vaginitis, with the Vulvitis. Clotrimazole, vaginal pessaries (500mg single dose, 200mg for three nights or 100mg for six nights) or, Clotrimazole cream (10% in a single 5gm application) or, Econazole pessary (150mg in a single dose, or repeated for three nights) or, Miconazole Ovule (1.2 gm in a single dose) or Miconazole pessary (200mg for seven nights) or Miconazole cream (2%, 5gm applications, daily for two weeks).

Oral therapy is preferred by patients who consider the topical applications messy. Oral therapy should be avoided during pregnancy or lactation. Oral preparations include: Fluconazole (50mg, in a single dose) or Itraconazole (200mg, twice daily for 1 day).

Recurrent vulvo-vaginal candidiasis patients may follow one of two approaches in the management. *Maintenance therapy* has the advantage of a respite but caries the disadvantage of recurrence in up to half of the patients after cessation of treatment. Fluconazole (100 mg orally, weekly) or Clotrinazole (500mg vaginal pessary, weekly) or Itraconazole (400mg, orally, once/month) could be used. *Episodic treatment* has the benefit of confirmed diagnosis and avoidance of over-treatment.

Male Patients: Partners of patients suffering with RVVC do not require treatment. There is no evidence that treatment of the male partner reduces recurrences. Patients suffering with Candidal Balanoposthitis benefit from saline lavage for the preputial sac; insuring rinse and dry conditions following the lavage. Moderate and severe Balanoposthitis require topical treatment; for example, Clotrimazole cream (2% twice daily), or Ketconazole cream (2%, twice daily). The Hydrocortisone containing antifungal preparations are valuable, when there is an element of hypersensitivity. They should not be used for extended periods or without medical supervision. The can conceal the diagnosis of an underlying and un- diagnosed dermatological condition (e.g., Balanitis Xerotica Obliterans). There are advantages for the patient to develop a habit of regular saline lavage of the preputial sac, on daily basis, which may eliminate or reduce recurrencies.

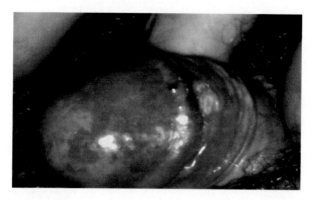

Figure 5. Severe Balanitis and bleeding

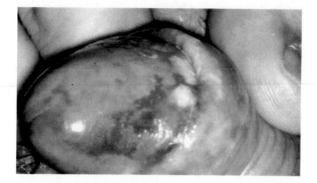

Figure 6. Balanitis associated with Penile Intra-Epithelial Neoplasia (PIN)

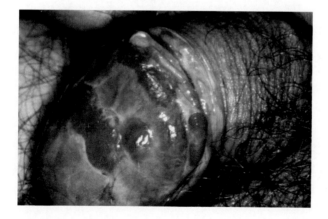

Figure 7. Severe Balanitis and erosions

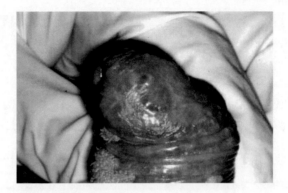

Figure 8. Balanitis associated with Warts

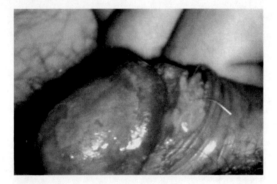

Figure 9. Candidal Balanitis

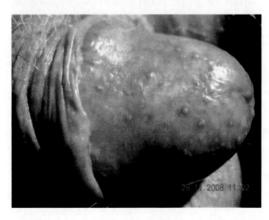

Figure 10. Candidal Balanitis

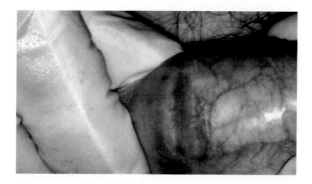

Figure 11. Localized Balanitis

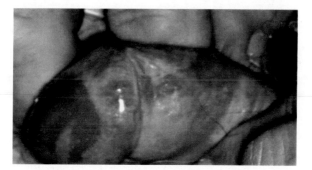

Figure 12. Lymphocytic Balanitis

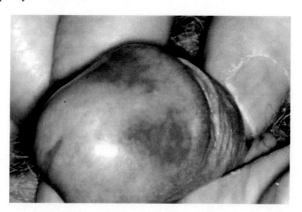

Figure 13. Lymphocytic Balanitis

Trichomoniasis

Trichomonas vaginalis is a flagellated oval protozoan, measuring 15 μm in length. The protozoan has five flagellae; four anterior that propel the organism, the fifth attached to an undulating membrane, that extend halfway the side of the organism. A central axostyle supports the organism and projects from its posterior end. The organism multiplies by mitosis, in 8-12 hours cycles. It contains large cytoplasmic granules for catabolism but has no mitochondria. It requires moist environment, temperature range of 35-37° C and acidic medium for growth. These conditions are usually available in the genito urinary tract. The organism is distributed world wide but is declining in western and industrialised countries; possibly due to the increasing recurrent use of antibiotics for concurrent conditions. The incidental identification of the protozoan on cervical cytology, followed by treatment, may contribute to diagnosis in asymptomatic cases. The organism is sexually- transmitted with the genital secretions. It could be retrieved from any cavity in the lower genital tracts of either females or males. The urinary flow may clear the organism from the male urethra; which decreases the chance of its retrieval with the time lapse between infection and testing. The anatomy of the female genital tract encourages the organism to thrive, for a longer period.

Clinical Presentation

Asymptomatic Trichomoniasis is common, affecting up to half of the infected female and male patients; when the organism is incidentally identified on testing. Female patients complain of vaginal discharge, Dysuria, Vulvo-Vaginal discomfort and/or burning. On examination, there is usually evidence of Vulvo-

Vaginitis. The typical discharge is profuse, thin, frothy and yellow. The discharge is occasionally, scanty and thick, as consequence of other concurrent infections. In severe conditions, there is evidence of cervical haemorrhagic punctations and ulcerations (strawberry cervix).

In males, the organism may be associated with Non-Gonococcal Urethritis (NGU). The patient may complain of discharge. The organism can cause Balanoposthitis, ulcerations and/or suppuration; and could be retrieved from the preputial sac. It is thought to be implicated with prostatitis

A sample of discharge, mixed with isotonic saline, examined by dark ground or phase contrast microscopy can give an immediate diagnosis. The organism has distinctive motility, with flagellae and undulating membrane. The tests have the advantage of immediate initiation of treatment. The organism is also identifiable on a dry smear, stained with acridine orange and examined by fluorescent microscopy. This requires laboratory, staff expertise and time; and is likely to delay initiation of treatment. The organism requires partial or complete anaerobic conditions for culture. Genital tract swabs and samples could be inoculated, directly into a culture medium, (e.g., Feinberg- Whittington Medium), or indirectly from a transport medium (e.g., Stuart's or Amies's). The process is laborious and many laboratories continue to depend on the wet preparation and microscopy tests. Latex agglutination and Polymerase Chain Reaction (PCR) give higher sensitivity and specificity; but are not available commercially yet.

Treatment

The first line of treatment is Metronidazole (400mg, orally, twice daily, for 7 days). A single dose regimen (2gm, orally) has the advantage of ensuring compliance; and is favoured by some patients; to avoid abstinence from alcohol intake. Tinidazole (2gm orally) provide an alternative.

Treatment of Resistant Trichomoniasis: Metronidazole (400mg, orally, three times daily, for 10 days) plus Erythromycin (250mg, orally, four times daily, for 7 days), or Amoxicillin (250mg, orally, three times daily, for 7 days).

Alternatively, Tinidazole (2gm, orally, twice daily) with Erythromycin (250 mg, orally, four times daily) and Clotrimazole vaginal pessaries (500mg daily), all for fourteen days.

Intravenous Metronidazole (3.5g daily for 14 days) is proposed as a therapeutic alternative in resistant cases but must be weighed against the patient's clinical condition.

Clinical Practicalities

1. A patient diagnosed with Trichomoniasis requires tests to exclude other concurrent STIs.
2. The patient requires systemic treatment as the organism may be present in the urethral and/or para-urethral pouches and cause re-infection.
3. The sex partner require simultaneous treatment
4. The couple should be advised on abstinence from sexual intercourse, to avoid re-infection, until treatment is completed.
5. The single dosage regimen may give the patient the false sense of security, of completed treatment and resumption of sexual intercourse, leading to re-infection.
6. Non-sexual transmission by fomites and sex toys may lead to shared infections between partners.
7. Vertical transmission may lead to Vulvo-Vaginitis in neonates, following acquisition during passage through infected maternal genital tract.
8. Trichomoniasis in a child, beyond the age of one should raise the possibility of sexual abuse.
9. In suspected treatment failures, re-infection from a sex partner should be excluded.
10. Metronidazole could be inactivated by mixed vaginal bacteria (e.g., β haemolytic Streptococci) which may lead to treatment failure. The addition of Erythromycin or Amoxicillin to Metronidazole may be necessary, to eliminate the inactivation effect of Streptococci.

Pediculosis

The causative organism is Pthirus pubis. The insect is 2 mm dark grey, with 3 claw-like legs on each side for attachment to the pubic hair. It has antennaethat are sensitive to human odour. It has tactile hairs. The female lays 2-3 eggs a day and 50 eggs during its lifetime. The eggs (nits) measure some 0.8mm and attach to the hair base, to facilitate accesses of the hatched nymphs to blood, from the hair follicle. Eggs hatch into nymphs in seven days and the life cycle (i.e., eggs, nits and adults) takes up to 25 days. The organism differs from body lice, which is larger and more oblong.

The incubation period range from 5 days to several weeks; allowing for the life cycle. Transmission is by skin-to-skin contact, hence the need for intimate contact and sexual acquisition The adult organism cannot live without host conditions for more than 2 days. Infestation from nits, included in bed linen and clothes, is likely. The patient may present with irritation in the genital skin and erythema; due to hypersensitivity reactions. The finding of insects and/or nits may be the presenting symptom.The coarse pubic hair is the usual site, but other body hair and eye lashes may be affected. The organism may affect other parts of the body, in hairy individuals (e.g., upper thigh, lower abdomen and/or chest). There may be evidence of insect activity in the form of red spots from host blood; or black spots from organism's faecal matter, in the underwear. The patient's skin may show 2-3 mm blue macules (Maculae Caeruleae), which is a reaction to the organism's saliva at the feeding site. The lesions are painless and do not fade on pressure.

The diagnosis is made on the clinical picture.Identifying the organism and/or eggs could be confirmed by low power microscopy.

The treatment options are topical application of Permethrin (1% aqueous lotion, applied to all body hair, for 12 hours, followed by a bath) or Permethrin (1% cream rinse, applied to damp hair, for 2 hours, followed by a rinse). The preparation could be used during pregnancy or lactation. Malathion (0.5% aqueous lotion) is an alternative, but not suitable during pregnancy or lactation. Infestation of eye lashes could be treated with Permethrin 1% lotion application for 10 minutes, with eyes closed for protection. Alternatively, insect suffocation could be achieved with the application of an inert ointment, twice daily for 10 days.

Clinical Practicalities

1. The patient should be advised on tests for other STIs.
2. Sex partner/s, for the previous three months, should be contact traced and offered assessment for pediculosis and other STIs.
3. The partners should be advised to abstain from sexual intercourse until the completion of both treatment courses.
4. The patient's clothes and bed linen need washing in high temperature. Items not suitable for washing, could be steam ironed.The aim is to destroy any nits or insects; to avoid reinfestation.

Scabies

Sarcopets scabiei is a mite that burrows into the stratum corneum of the skin, up to 5 mm per day, to lay eggs. The adult organism is slightly oblong (0.3 x 0.4mm), and have 8 legs. Adults lay up to 3 eggs daily. The eggs hatch into larvae, in 4 days. The larvae develop into nymphs, then to adults. The life cycle is 10 days and the life span is 6 weeks Males demise after mating.

Transmission takes place by skin to skin contact. Holding hands is the most likely route of transmission and requires prolonged contact (i.e., a hand shake or a short hug is not a likely cause of infestation). Scabies could be a family infestation and can cause outbreaks in schools, nurseries and nursing homes.

The patient usually presents with intense irritation, especially at night, due to immunological response to mite excrements. The primary attack may be asymptomatic initially; until the patient mounts an immunological reaction, some 6 weeks' later. Secondary infestations become symptomatic within a day or two. The lesions are eczematous, with papules, vesicles, and/or nodules, especially on genital skin. The lesions are burrows appearing as silvery lines; affecting hands, finger webs, wrists, axillae, extensor aspect of elbows, genitals and/or buttocks. In female patients, the areas around the nipples could be affected. Secondary infestations may follow scratching and auto-inoculation; transmitting the insect from one part of the body to another.

Diagnosis is mostly clinical. It is possible to identify the burrows by the application of washable ink to the suspected llesion; which fills the burrow and remains after washing the ink. Topical Tetracycline applied to the site will also fill the burrow and fluoresce under Wood's light. It may be possible to retrieve the mites, from burrows, with a needle for microscopic inspection. There is good treatment response to Permethrin (5% cream), Malathion (0.5% aqueous lotion) or Benzyl benzoate. It is advisable to repeat the treatment after one week.

Crusted Scabies (Norwegian Scabies): The classical infestation with scabies involves 5-10 mites. In patients with reduced immune response, the reduced sensitisation and, consequently lack of symptoms, leads to unlimited multiplication and, consequently, infestation with thousands of mites. It affects the immuno-compromised individuals (e.g., patients with HIV or under chemotherapy) or frail persons. The condition is highly contagious. It is clinically identified by crustations, hyperkeratotic lesions and honeycombed cavities. It is essential to repeat treatment, if topical preparations are used. Ivermectin (200µg/kg orally as a single dose) could be added, if there is no response to topical therapy. Household contacts may require treatment.

Clinical Practicalities

1. The infestation requires close contact, hence sexual transmission.
2. The patient should be offered tests to exclude other STIs.
3. The sex partner should be assessed
4. Both partners should be advised to abstain from close contact, until both complete the treatment.
5. Skin irritation and itching may continue for several weeks following treatment and could be helped with antihistaminics.
6. Clothes and bedding need washing in high temperature.
7. Sexual and intimate contacts, for the previous 3 months, should be traced.

Sexually Transmitted Viral Hepatitis

Hepatitis A Virus (HAV) Infection

Hepatitis A virus (HVA) infection is caused by a picorna (RNA) virus. The virus has a world-wide distribution; and is more prevalent in areas with poor sanitation. Transmission is faeco-oral (i.e by food and/or water, contaminated with infected faeces or urine), or close personal contacts (e.g., oro-genital and oro-anal sexual practices). High risk groups are men having sex with men and persons with multiple sexual partners. There is evidence of transmission by contaminated blood products.

The incubation period is 2-6 weeks and the disease may progress unnoticed. Most of the children and half of the adults are either asymptomatic or suffer non-specific complaints. The icteric illness lasts up to 3 weeks, but may extend to 12 weeks with Cholestasis. The patient may present with jaundice, upper abdominal symptoms and pain. A prodromal phase, of flu-like illness, that existed for 3-10 days and improved at the onset of jaundice, could be recognised in retrospect.

The clinical signs are non-specific in the prodromal phase. The icteric phase is marked with jaundice, pale stools and dark urine, slight hepatic enlargement and tenderness. One in ten patients may require hospital care and fulminating hepatitis complicates approximately 4 in 1000. Liver function tests project the picture of hepatic and cholestatic jaundice. Hepatitis A may affect patients already infected with Hepatitis B or C. HAV during pregnancy can lead to early abortion, prematurity and/or HAV vertical transmission. HAV specific IgM help the diagnosis and confirmation; whilst IgG indicates previous exposure or vaccination.

The condition could be managed on an out patient basis, with rest and oral hydration. Hospitalisation is required in a minority of cases, where there are signs of dehydration and/or hepatic decompensation.

Clinical Practicalities

1. The patient should be advised to avoid sexual intercourse or handling food until clearance of the acute phase and confirmation of no infectivity.
2. The patient should be assessed for other STIs, if sexual transmission is considered, with contact tracing and assessment of sexual contacts.
3. Contacts, who run risk of contamination through food or water, should be considered for HVA assessement.

Hepatitis B Virus (HBV) Infection

Hepatitis B virus (HBV) is caused by a Hepadna (DNA) Virus. Six genotypes (A-F) have been identified. Hepatitis B is endemic worldwide, with a carriage rate reaching 20%. The rate in the UK is 1-4:10,000 individuals. The unscrupulous use of contaminated syringes/needles contributes to the high parenteral transmission in some communities. Contaminated blood, blood products are also a factor. Vertical transmission from mother to child contributes to high prevalence in the Far East. Sexual transmission is higher with oro-anal and receptive rectal than vaginal sex. Healthcare professionals are at risk of infection by transmission from infected patients and/or carriers.

The incubation period ranges from 6 weeks to 6 months. The condition may progress unnoticed. Most of the infected infants and children and up to 50% of adults are asymptomatic. In symptomatic cases, the prodromal and icteric phases are similar to Hepatitis A, but may be severe and prolonged, especially in HIV patients who are likely to be symptomatic. Acute infection carries a risk of mortality, from fulminating Hepatitis, of 1 in 100. Chronicity is defined by the persistence of the surface antigen (HBsAg) and affects 1 in 10 patients. Chronicity is higher in patients with HIV, immuno-compromise, chronic renal failure or immunosuppressive therapy. Up to 50% of chronic carriers will develop cirrhosis; which is higher with concurrent HIV infection. Ten percent of cirrhosis patients will develop liver cancer; which is higher with concurrent Hepatitis C infection. Pregnant women carry the risk of early aportion, premature delivery and vertical transmission.

Clinical Practicalities

1. Hepatitis A and/or B vaccination is valuable only after early exposure, possibly up to 7 days.
2. Human immunoglobulin should be considered early after exposure. The diagnosis of the index case takes place at the icteric phase; which reduces the practicality of early treatment with human immunoglobulin.
3. Prophylactic immunisation of at-risk groups (e.g., homosexuals and/or HIV patients) with combined Hepatitis A and B vaccine should be considered.
4. There will be patients in this group who will not respond to Hepatitis B vaccination, possibly due to impaired immunity.
5. Hepatitis A and B vaccination is advisable before travel to a high prevalence area and at risk homosexual men.
6. Immunity is usually life-long, following Hepatitis A exposure or vaccination. For Hepatitis B, Booster dosages are required; timed by levels of antibodies.
7. The mainstay of prevention is health education on routes of transmission and avoidance of contamination
8. Breast feeding should not be prohibited.

Hepatitis C Virus (HCV) Infection

Hepatitis C virus (HCV) is caused by RNA virus; and is endemic worldwide. There are 7 known subtypes of HCV. The prevalence in UK varies from 6:10,000 blood donors to 6:10 intravenous drug users (IVDUs). Sexual transmission is rare and is higher in HIV infected patients. The majority of infections are parenteral (i.e., IVDUs, transfusion of contaminated blood or blood products and infected sharps). The denial of HCV infected individuals of any risk factors compromises the identification of the exact route of transmission.

The incubation period varies and may extend to 20 weeks. HCV antibodies usually develop after 3 months, take longer in some patients and may not develop at all in a number of cases. The infection is asymptomatic in most of the patients. It is uncommon to have icteric Hepatitis. Fulminating Hepatitis is rare, affecting less than 1% and higher with concurrent Hepatitis A infection. Up to 80% of the patients become carriers and mortality is very low in the acute phase. Thirty percent of chronic carriers will progress to severe liver disease; which may take up to 20 years to develop. One in three patients caries the risk of developing cirrhosis and one in twenty may develop liver cancer.

Diagnosis could be confirmed within 2 weeks of infection, by HCV-RNA. HCV antibody tests are used for screening. There is a window period of 3 months; and could be longer in a number of patients. The persistence of HCV-RNA beyond 6 months identifies chronicity. HCV genotyping helps to plane prognosis and response to therapy.

Treatment in the acute icteric phase is similar to Hepatitis A. There are indications that alpha interferon can reduce chronicity. Pegylated Interferon Alpha, weekly subcutaneous injections; and Ribavirin, daily twice oral dosages, can abolish chronicity. The treatment requires monitoring. The response is better in genotypes 2 and 3. Genotypes 1, 4, 5 or 6 should be tested for response after 12 weeks of therapy; and the treatment is continued for those expressing evidence of response. Co-infection with HIV reduces response to treatment.

Clinical Practicalities

1. Hepatitis C acute condition is a notifiable disease in the UK.
2. The patient and HIV infected sex partner/s should be advised on the possibility of sexual transmission and the long-term health consequences.
3. Hepatitis C patients benefit from vaccination against Hepatitis A and B, as co-infections can lead to Fulminating Hepatitis.
4. There is no available vaccine or immunoglobulin that will prevent transmission.
5. There is evidence of vertical transmission, but not through breastfeeding.
6. The patient is not suitable for donating blood, semen or organs.

Hepatitis D Virus (HDV) Infection

Hepatitis D virus (HDV) is incomplete RNA and requires the outer coat of Hepatitis B Virus. HDV is found only in patients with HBV. The risk population are IVDUs, their sexual partners, and female sex workers. It should be suspected in Hepatitis B patients with severe acute condition, rapidly progressive chronic HBV or with superimposed acute episodes. It carries a higher risk of fulmination and chronicity. Diagnosis is made by identifying HDV antibodies or RNA. There is no valuable antiviral therapy for HDV.

Tropical Sexually Transmitted Infections

Chancroid

Chancroid is caused by Haemophilus ducreyi, a Gram negative cocco-bacillus, found in chains. Its culture requires moisture, blood enriched material and 10% carbon dioxide atmosphere for incubation. It is the most common cause of Genital Ulcerative Disease (GUD) in developing countries, accounting for 1 in 3 cases of STIs in Africa. Prostitutes are important reservoirs ; due to the non-symptomatic carriage of H ducreyi.

The incubation period ranges from 1 to 14 days. Infection requires intimate sexual contact; including oral sex. The organism could be transmitted by Auto-inoculation. The lesions start with a papule, leading to pustule, then ulcer formation. The ulcer is about 2 cm in diameter, has an irregular margin and bleeds on touch. Its base is not indurated. Multiple ulcerations may coalesce into a giant ulcer. The ulcers are genital, may affect any part; but have predilection to folds (e.g., preputial sac or inbetween vulval lips). Homosexual patients, recipients of rectal sex, develop anal lesions. The inguinal lymph nodes swell and become tender and may develop abscess (bubon). Extra genital lesions may affect the breasts or fingers. The ulcers may be complicated with super-imposed secodery infection, leading to excessive tissue destruction (phagedenic chancroid); or inguinal sinus.

Diagnosis is made by microscopy of Gram-stained smear, of material obtained from the ulcer, after its cleansing. Culture is diagnostic but may give false negative result in 1 in 4 cases. EIA and PCR tests are not commercially available.

The therapeutic options include Ciprofloxacin (500 mg, orally, twice daily for three days), or Azithromycin (1g, orally, in a single dose), or Ceftriaxone (250mg, intra-muscularly, in a single dosage) or Erythromycin (500mg, orally, four times daily for seven days). Fluctuating inguinal lymph nodes and abscesses require aspiration, to release pressure. The options should consider drugs that are not anti-treponemal, to avoid masking concurrent syphilitic conditions. Sex partner/s, within 10 days of the first symptoms in the index case, should be traced for assessment and treatment.

Lymphogranuloma venereum (LGV)

Lymphogranuloma venereum (LGV) is caused by Chlamydia trachomatis serovars L1, L2 and L3. It is widespread in tropical and sub-tropical areas across the globe. It is usually sexually transmitted and associated with lower social conditions, multiplicity of sexual partners and prostitution. All sexual practices are implicated, including use of sex toys. Cases of LGV in homosexual males and HIV patients, were identified in patients with history of sexual networks and group sex. Asymptomatic nature of the condition, in some patients, promotes propagation.

Primary Lympho-granuloma venereum has an incubation period of few days to a month. The lesions start with a papule at the site of inoculation, changing to pustule then ulcer. LGV affect any part of the genitalia; with predilection to folds; and may affect the mouth.

Secondary Lympho-granuloma venereum takes place after a week to six months following the primary infection. The patient may develop systemic inflammatory conditions; namely arthritis, meningitis, peri-hepatitis, pneumonia, erythema nodosum and/or erythema multiforme. The relevant lymph nodes are affected (e.g., inguinal, femoral or pelvic); but their enlargement may be concealed (e.g., in pelvic lymph-adenopathy).

Tertiary Lympho-granuloma venereum leads to porcto-colitis. The patient presents with rectal discharge, bleeding, tenesmus, fever and malaise. In chronic conditions abscesses, constrictions, scarring and fistula may develop. Chronic lymphatic involvement leads to inflammation, sclerosis and obstruction. It can lead to localised oedema (e.g., Saxophone penis); or generalised oedema and eventually Genital Elephantiasis.

Diagnosis is confirmed with LGV complement fixation test, in the presence of the clinical features. A four-fold increase in antibody level, or a titre of 1:64 or more, support the diagnosis. Cell culture for C trachomatis requires special laboratory conditions. The culture has a false negative rate of 20%. The Nucleic Acid Amplification Test (NAAT) is sensitive but is not licensed for anal, rectal and oro-pharyngeal samples. Outbreaks of LGV in Western Europe, during 2003 and 2004, have led to the development of a public health laboratory enhanced surveillance programme in the UK.

Treatment options include Doxycycline (100mg, orally, twice daily for three weeks) or Erythromycin (500mg, orally, four times daily for three weeks). The Dutch clinical experience suggests good response to Azithromycin (1g orally in a single dose). The sex partner/s should be traced for assessment for LGV between other STIs. There is a place for the initiation of epidemiological treatment, after taking samples for tests.

Donovanosis (Granuloma inguinale)

Donovanosis is a sexually transmitted condition leading to genital ulceration. The causative organism is a Gram negative pleomorphic bacterium: Klebsiella (Calymmatobacterium) granulomatise. The rarity of the condition in the sex partners of patients with open lesions casts doubt on exclusive sexual transmission. Non-sexual transmission, with direct inoculation from contaminated skin or faeces, carries risk to young children and healthcare workers. The incubation period is usually four weeks and may extend to a year. The organism prefers moist mucous and muco-cutaneous areas. Lesions start with a papule, then a nodule or a plaque, breaking into an ulcer, at the site of inoculation. The nodules are caused by granulomatous formation and may reach 2 cm in diameter. Necrosis can lead to scarring; distortion of the overlying tissue or stenosis of encircled organs (e.g., anus, vagina and/or urethra). Haematogenous spread may take place and effect distant organs, viscera and/or bone; presenting in some cases as abscesses. Regional lymph nodes enlarge, develop abscesses and may be complicated with secondary bacterial infection. Lymphatic involvement may lead to genital oedema (e.g., Genital Elephantiasis).

Dignosis is confirmed on the identification of Donovan Bodies. They are Gram negative, bipolar and pleomorphic appearance, measuring 2x0.7μm and has a visible capsule; located within a large mono-nuclear leucocytes. Cellular material may be obtained by biopsy, stained with silver stain, or scraping the lesion/ulcer, stained with Giemsa stain. Cell culture and polymerase chain reactions (PCR) tests are available for research.

Treatment options include Azithromycin (1g orally, weekly for 6 weeks or 500mg daily for seven days) or Doxycycline (100mg orally, twice daily, for three weeks) or Ciprofloxacin (750mg orally, twice daily, for three weeks). Treatment should continue, if there is evidence of unhealed lesion and until full resolution. Streptomycin, Chloramphenicol and Oxytetracycline have a record of effectiveness; and may be considered in cases of drug allergies to the first line choices.

During pregnancy, Erythromycin (500mg orally, four times daily for three weeks) could be used. Vertical transmission is possible, due to infection from untreated genital lesions and requires consideration of prophylactic antibiotics for the neonate.

The sex partner/s should be traced, for assessment and treatment.

Sexually Acquired Reactive Arthritis (SARA)

Sexually Acquired Reactive Arthritis (SARA) is sero-negative sterile inflammation of the synovial membrane, tendons and fascia, triggered by STI. The association of SARA with HIV disease is higher in Africans.

Active arthritis associated with urethritis and conjunctivitis is referred to as Reiter's Syndrome; which may or may not be associated with cutaneous or mucous-membrane lesions. SARA presents in males 2-4 weeks after urethritis (NGU). It is less common in females; when cervicitis is likely to be unrecognised. The mechanism and relationship between infection and SARA is not clear. Chlamydia trachomatis, Ureaplasma urealyticum and Mycoplasma genitalium DNA had been identified in the synovial fluid of some patients with SARA. The association with other uro-genital infections has been reported, in 30 to 70% of patients, according to different studies. N gonorrhoca, apart from causing septic arthritis, is implicated in SARA. Other enteric infections (e.g., Salmonella and Shigella), can cause reactive arthritis. Human Leucocyte Antigen B27 (HLA – B27) positivity is prognostic of chronicity and recurrences; and suggest 50-folds increased risk for developing SARA.

The clinical features are mainly of symmetrical polyarthritis; with predominance to the lower limbs and appearing 2 weeks after uro-genital infections. The loss of muscle bulk, in relation to affected joints, could be rapid. Scro-iliac, lower lumbar and sacral vertebral joints are affected. Inflammation involves the insertion point of ligaments, tendons and capsules. Most cases are associated with urethritis in males or urethritis and/or cervicitis in females. Some patients may have evidence of cystitis and rarely glomerulo-nephritis. Ophthalmic complications include conjunctivitis, iritis, keratitis and/or episcleritis. Muco-cutaneous changes are widespread and variable. Lesions may take the form of Pustular Psoriasis. These may be localized, affecting soles and/or palms, or generalised (Keratoderma Blennorrhagica). Circumcised men may develop psoriasis like balanitis. The uncircumcised, may develop erythematous patches with well-defined margins in a geographical appearance (Circinate Balanitis). Oral lesions, in the form of erythematous patches, ulcerations or geographical tongue affect 1 in 10 patients. The general manifestations may include myocarditis, pericarditis, aortitis, pleurisy, meningo-encephalitis, peripheral neuropathies, optic neuritis and/or enterocolitis.

The disease is self-limiting in most cases, with 50% recurrences. HLA - B27 genetyping helps in determining disease course and prognosis. The first episode may extend to 6 months. One in 5 patients may develop chronic symptoms. The mainstay of diagnosis is the clinical picture of SARA, the identification of genito-urinary infection/ inflammation and the presence of sero-negative active arthritis. Rest and non-steroidal anti-inflammatory drugs (NSAIDs), physiotherapy and physical therapy are called upon in response to the clinical picture. Cyclo-oxygenase (COX) 2 selective drugs have the advantage of low gastrointestinal complications. Alternatively, gastro-protective agents (e.g., Proton pump inhibitor, Histamine-2 blockers or Misoprostol) reduce NSAIDs risks. The usual regimens are advisable. There is no evidence of benefits from longer courses or higher dosages. The assistance of other specialists (e.g., rheumatologists, neurologists and/or ophthalmologists) should be timely sought. Complicated and prolonged cases of SARA are better dealt with by a team of clinicians acquainted with disabling joint conditions. Antibiotic therapy should be used for the treatment of concurrent genito-urinary infection. Intra-articular corticosteroid injections may have benefits in some cases. Systemic corticosteroids, Sulphasalazine and Methotrexate have a place, if the condition is disabling. Azathioprine, gold salts, D Penicillamine and Tumour Necrosis Factors (TNF) α blockers may be required.

Practical Considerations

1. Visual/Eye symptoms should benefit from a slit lamp assessment, to diagnosis or exclude uveitis. Untreated uveitis may result in visual loss and early ophthalmological advice should be sought.
2. The patient should be advised to avoid triggering infections (e.g., STIs).

3. Extra genital manifestations are better managed by the relevant specialists.

Syphilis

The name "Syphilis" was introduced by an Italian physician and poet, who presented an epic of a shepherd named Syphilis. The physician carried the name and used it in his medical writings "On Contagious Diseases". The condition has also been called the French Disease, Cupid's Disease and Great Pox.

The Organism

The disease is caused by Treponema pallidum which has four sub-species: T pallidum pallidum, causing Syphilis, T pallidum pertenue which causes Yaws, T pallidum carateum which causes Pinta; and T pallidum endemicum which causes Bejel. The organism is a spirochaete, measuring up to 20 μm X 0.18 μm. It contains a nucleus, cytoplasm and surrounded with a protein envelope. It does not survive outside the human body, hence the need of intimate contact and sexual transmission. The other Treponemal sub-species are similar in morphology and serology tests to T pallidum; therefore are difficult to distinguish in clinical practice. They are not transmitted through sexual contact and have a different disease pattern.

Prevalence

The WHO estimated that 12 million new cases of Syphilis were acquired during 1999; 4 million in South East Asia, 4 million in Africa and 3 million in South America. In some underdeveloped countries, up to 15% of women of childbearing age have Syphilis. One in three pregnant women with Syphilis will have still-birth and one in three will have a neonate with congenital Syphilis; which has a mortality of up to 50%.

The US CDC reported 36,000 cases of Syphilis in 2006, half of whom were aged 20 to 39; and 349 cases of Congenital Syphilis. The UK Health Protection Agency received reports of 2,766 cases of syphilis in 2006; an increase of 1,607% since 1997. Outbreaks in the UK and other European countries are remarkable in men who have sex with men.

Clinical Presentation

Transmission

Syphilis is transmitted by close contact, helped by moisture and trauma to mucous/cutaneous surfaces. Genital transmission is the most common route. The vulnerability of the organism to heat and desiccation, makes transmission almost exclusively venereal. Primary and secondary stage lesions are highly contagious and infectious. The most infectious stage is Early Syphilis, with half of the contacts acquiring the infection. The incubation period ranges from 9-90 days, usually between 18-28 days, after infection.

Secondary stage body fluids, semen, saliva and/or blood remain infective, for up to 2 years and occasionally longer. Oro-genital transmission is commoner in homosexuals. Trans-placental transmission, from an infected mother, is high in Early Syphilis. Vertical transmission takes place between infected untreated mothers and the infant, by direct contact. There is a risk of transmission through sharing needles (e.g., intravenous drug users) and accidental inoculation (e.g., health care workers); but requires fresh samples and large innoculum.

Early Syphilis

After inoculation, the organism is carried to the regional lymph nodes within the first 24hrs and possibly within few minutes. Lesions of primary syphilis take place at the site of infection. The typical clinical presentation of early syphilis is painless papule that expands and ulcerates producing a chancre; 1-2cm in diameter with indurated margin and moist base. The lesion appears at the site of inoculation; most likely the mucosal surface of the genitalia. Oral, anal and rectal lesions are associated with oral and anal sex. Intra-lumenal (e.g., rectal) lesion may be concealed and go unnoticed by the patient. Any part of the human tegumemt, with a breach of its integrity, could be an entrance, leading to a primary lesion (*Chancre*). Extra-genital lesions (eg. fingers, hands, nipples) may result from contact with an infectious lesion. Historical records have examples of almost in any part of the body affected by Chancres. They may be single or multiple. Chancres may not arise, if the innoculum is small, or concealed by skin folds. The chancre is usually associated with painless enlargement of the regional lymph nodes; described as hard, non-tender and rubbery. The primary lesion may be atypical, in the form of Balanitis (Syphilitic Balanitis of Follman), or multiple ulcers associated with secondary infection, pain and resembling genital herpes. Atypical lesions require vigilant clinical awareness and attention. In the presence of secondary infection, the lymph nodes may be tender.

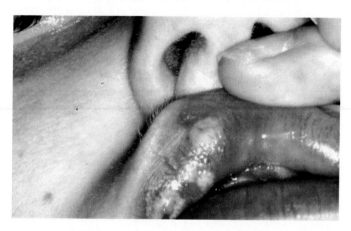

Figure 1. Secondery Syphilis: Lip Condyloma and mucous patches

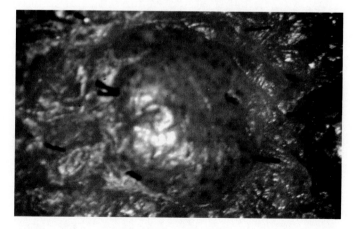

Figure 2. Secondery Syphilis: Nipple Condyloma

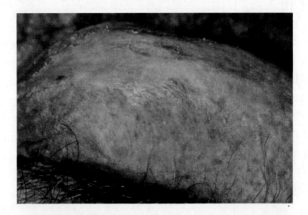

Figure 3. Secondary Syphilitic Penile Rash

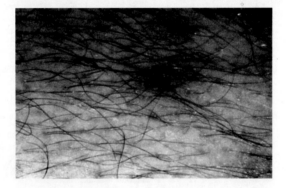

Figure 4. Secondary Syphilitic Body Rash

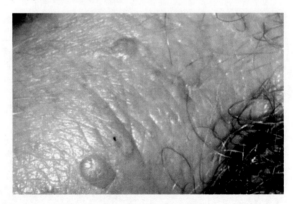

Figure 5. Secondary Syphilitic Penile Papules/ Macules

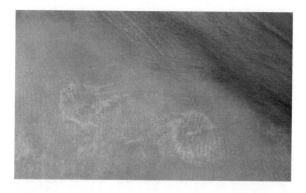

Figure 6. Secondary Syphilis: Annular Rash

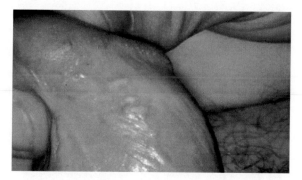

Figure 7. Secondary Syphilis: Penile Papules

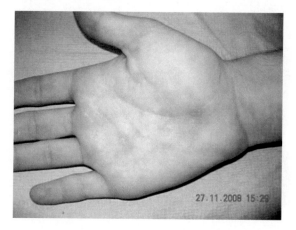

Figure 8. Secondary Syphilitic Palm Rash

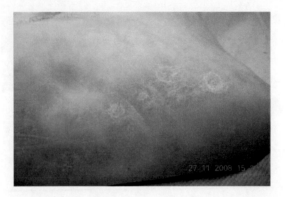

Figure 9. Secondary Syphilitic Annular Rash

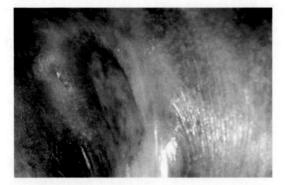

Figure 10. Syphilitic Balanitis

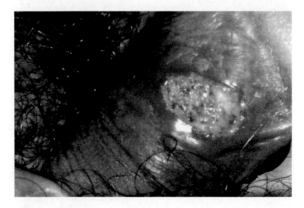

Figure 11. Syphilitic Penile Ulcerative Chancre

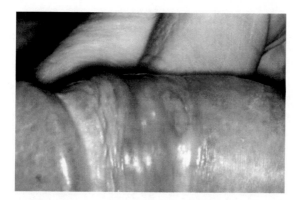

Figure 12. Syphilitic Penile Ulcer

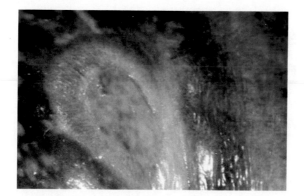

Figure 13. Syphilitic Penile Ulcer

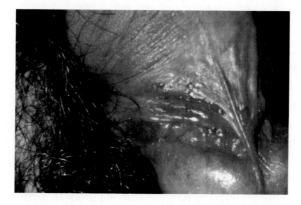

Figure 14. Syphilitic Penile Ulcer

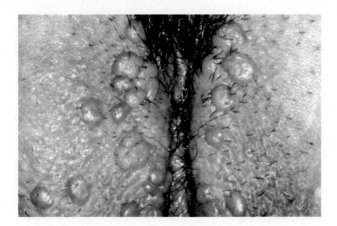

Figure 15. Vulval/Perineal Condylomata Lata

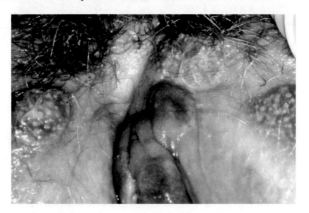

Figure 16. Vulval Condylomata Lata

Secondary Syphilis

Secondary syphilis may take place 1-6 months after infection; usually 6-8 weeks. Haematogenous dissemination leads to fever, headache, malaise and myalgia. The most common manifestations of secondary syphilis are generalised rash and adenitis. Mucous patches and Condylomata Lata are less common. The less common manifestations of secondary syphilis deserve clinical attention in the process of differential diagnosis.

The skin rash (Syphilides) is polymorphic and may take any form, macular, maculo-pappular, anullar, circinate or pustulo-ulcerative. The palms and soles are commonly affected. There is generalised Lymph-adenopathy; and the primary stage lymph nodes could possibly remain enlarged. There may be leukoderma (e.g., of the neck). The rash could rarely be vesicular, pustular or Itchy. Pustular rash can rarely occour in debilitating conditions. There may be patchy or diffused loss of hair (Moth-eaten Alopecia). Nail effects include change in pigmentation, pitting, brittleness and paronychia. Papules in moist areas (e.g., genital, anal, angle of mouth, under breasts, axially and/or between toes) produce flat, warty lesions (Condylomata Lata). Mucous membrane lesions may start with patches that ulcerate and may coalesce forming "snail-track ulcers". In the oro-pharyngeal cavity, the lesion may present as sore throat, in the laryngeal area as hoarseness of voice, in the nasal mucosa as discharge, and in the rectum as Proctitis. There could be remains of the primary lesion (Chancre), its scar or its history. The differential diagnosis of secondry syphilitic rash include drug reactions, psoriasis, Lichen planus, Pitryiasis rosea, Tinea versicolor, Infectious mononucleosis, measles and rubella.

Involvement of basal meningees may present with occipital headach. Optic neuritis may present as papilloedema and eight nerve effects as tinnitus. Iritis, anterior uveitis and optic nerve atrophy may take place. The manifestations may affect different organs causing hepatitis, nephritis, nephritic syndrome, arthritis, peri-ostitiis and/or peripheral neuritis. Secondary relapses of muco-cutaneous lesions may take place during the consecutive 2-4 years. In case of non-treatment, secondary stage lesions may take weeks or months, up to 9 months, to heal.

Latent Syphilis

Latent Syphilis identifies the condition of positive serology, with no clinical symptoms or signs; when the treponemes lie dormant in lymph nodes. The period of latent syphilis is identified in the UK after the first two years following infection; (one year in the USA and 1-4 years in other countries). When the point of sexual contact and acquisition is identifiable, it could be sub-divided into early latent (first two years) or late latent (more than two years).

Tertiary Syphilis

Tertiary Syphilis refers to late symptomatic stage but excluding meningo-vascular disease. Studies of untreated syphilis in Oslo in the earlier part of the 20th Centuary indicate that one third of the cases progress to a disease burn out, with spontaneous cure; but remaining positive tests for treponemal antigens and negative tests for non-treponemal antigens. In another third, there continued to be positivity for treponemal and non-treponemal antigen tests, but no clinical manifestations. The remaining third of patients develop tertiary complications and become symptomatic in late syphilis. One third, of the later group, develop gummata and the other two thirds, of late symptomatic syphilis, may develop cardio-vascular and/or neuro syphilis. A recent review of the Oslo group of untreated syphilis, calculates that Gumma formation takes place in 16%, cardio-vascular syphilis 10% and neurosyphilis in 7%.

Gummatous syphilis may develop in some 10-15 % of infected patients; usually 3-7 years later; but may be as late as 20 years or more. The lesion is a chronic inflammatory response to the organism, and results in an infiltrate of inflammatory cells, lymphocytes, plasma cells and epitheliod cells; followed by tissue necrosis and surrounded by fibrosis. It is usually single and golf ball in size. Multiple small and microscopic lesions were described. It may present as a space occupying lesion (e.g., in internal organs, brain, liver and/or muscle). When near the surface, it may ulcerate; but it is not contagious. The typical gummatous skin ulcer has a punched out edge. Multiple skin gummata, in different stages of development, lead to a mixture of nodulo- ulcerative lesions; with different stages of nodules, ulcerations and healing. Healed lesions have a tissue paper like thin scare.

Oral, nasal, pharyngeal gummata may affect any part of the tongue, lips, hard and soft palate, tonsillar fossae and/or posterior pharyngeal wall. It can lead to destruction of the effected part (eg. perforation of the nasal septum or destruction of the palate, which could be extensive and widespread). It may cause enlargement of the affected part, leading to macro-glossia or Leukoplakia, of lips, tongue and/or buccal mucosa. Gumma of the larynx may present as hoarseness of voice.

Early lung lesions could be confused with neoplasm and/or tuberculosis. Gastro-intestinal lesions may be localized, in the form of gumma or diffused in the form of fibrosis and its effects. It can lead to localised liver space-occupying lesion or diffused hepatic fibrosis. Extensive fibrosis can lead to lobulation of the liver (Hepar Lobatum). Diffused fibrosis in the liver may lead to portal obstruction, ascites and jaundice. Gummata of the kidneys, bladder and /or testicles are rare.

Bone lesions of late syphilis may affect the periosteal tissue; in the form of bone formation and/or destruction. Granulation tissue leads to bone formation and thickening of the pariosteal area. Bone destruction may extend inward (worm-eaten bones). Endosteal changes are gummatous and could ulcerate (e.g., palate and skull bones). Osseous changes are associated with local pain and tenderness; which is worse at night. It is more common in long bones but the skull, sternum and/or clavicles may be affected. Gummata are less common in communities where antibiotic use, for other concurrent non STI infections, is frequent and widespread.

The organism invades the CNS in 1 in 5 cases during the early stages of infection. In the absence of treatment half of these cases develop *neuro-syphilis*. Connective tissue and blood vessels involvement leads to *meningo-vascular syphilis;* which appear 3-7 years after infection. It may affect cerebral and/or spinal meninges. Cerebral meningo-vascular syphilis can lead to cranial nerve palsies and/or internal hydrocephalous. The patient may present with dizziness, vertigo, headache, blurred vision, diplopia, tinnitus and/or deafness. Vascular syphilis, due to endarteritis obliterans, can lead to narrowing of cerebral arteries, thrombosis and cerebral infarcts. The clinician should consider the exclusion of syphilis associated cerebro- vascular accidents in young adults (e.g., hemiplegia, hemianopia, vertigo, or mental decline). Spinal meningo-vascular syphilis may affect the anterior nerve roots; leading to muscle flaccidity, paralysis and atrophy. When the posterior roots are affected, there is sensory disruptions and pain. Autonomic nerve effects may lead to impotence, constipation and ortho-static hypotension. Loss of bladder sensation leads to retention and overflow incontinence. Spino-vascular accidents result in sudden paralysis, below the level of the lesion. There could be a mixed picture of cerebro-spinal and meningo-vascular syphilis

Occular syphilis may present with optic atrophy and/or opthalmoplegia; leading to visual disturbances, progressive loss of vision and ptosis. The typical small, irregular, unequal pupils; with constriction in response to accommodation but not to light (Argyl-Robertson Pupil), is diagnostic. Choroido-retinitis and interstitial keratitis may lead the clinical suspicion, which should be confirmed on serology tests. Iritis, chroidoretinitis and/or corneal ulcers may also occur.

CNS Parenchymal involvement may affect the brain and/or spinal cord. Syphilitic encephalitis can lead to diverse motor, sensory and psychiatric symptoms. There is a mixed picture of neural cell and fibre degeneration (ie. Parenchymal degeneration) cerebral atrophy, with fibrosis/gliosis and lymphocyte and plasma cell infiltrates. It could be associated with meningeal and vascular inflammation (i.e., a mixed picture of meningo-encephalitis). The patient may present with headache, loss of concentration, memory loss, personality changes, hallucinations and/or delusions. Bouts of mania and permanent paralysis gives the the name *"General Paralysis of the Insane"(GPI)* and "dementia paralytica". The condition presents 1-30 years after the infection, usually 10-20. There could be epileptic seizures A mixed and ameliorated picture of the above conditions may appear with incomplete treatment (e.g., antibiotic treatment for an incidental condition).

Degeneration and gross demyalination of the lumbo-sacral and lower thoracic dorsal root ganglia and spinal nerves, lead to loco-motor ataxia (*Tapes Dorsalis*). The condition appears 10-20 years after infection. Deep sensory loss leads to penetrating ulcers. Frequent trauma to joints, due to loss of deep sensation, leads to its destruction (*Charcot's joints*). The patient presents with paraethesiae, lightening pains, complaints of pins and needles, burning, stabbing or feeling of electric shocks, appearing in bouts, usually in the lower extremities. Similar symptoms in the gastric area may simulate acute surgical emergencies (e.g., abdominal pain and vomiting). In the laryngeal area, it may present with episodes of stridors or dyspnoea. Tabes Dorsalis and GPI are more common in males and Caucasians.

Gumma of the brain and/or spinal cord are rare. The clinical findings are: ataxia in the dark (Romberg sign), hypo-aethesia, absent cremasteric reflex, muscle/tendon areflexia and hypotonia, reduced sense of deep pain, loss of vibration sense, loss of joint position sense and flexor plantar reflex.

Cardio-vascular syphilis develops some 10-40 years following the infection, usually within 20 years. Syphilis affects small blood vessels that supply the aorta leading to a cscade of inflammation, destruction and fibrosis. This makes the aorta vulnerable to internal pressure, leading to aneurismal dilatation. The commonest part involved is the ascending aorta, pressing forward and displacing the trachea. In the aortic arch, the aneurysm compresses surrounding organs, leading to dysphagia, cough, stridors and hoarseness of voice. The effect on the aorta at the coronary osteae, can lead to their narrowing and cardiac ischaemia. There is risk of increased coronary osteal narrowing following antibiotic treatment; leading to acute coronary ischaemia and sudden death. The cardiac ischaemia could be perpetuated by coronary arteries atheroma. Aneurysmal dilatation at aortic valve level leads to aortic incompetence and regurgitation. Occasionally the aortic valve cusps' edges and attachment are involved with the syphilitic process and contributes to regurgitation. Aneurysmal dilatation of the whole descending thoracic aorta is usually asymptomatic; except for the aortic regurgitation. A saccular localised protrusion of the aorta may rupture, leading to fatal haemorrhage or severe bleeding to surrounding cavities/organs. Simple uncomplicated syphilitic aortitis was common before the antibiotic era. It presents with dull retro-sternal ache, that is not associated with exercise.There linear calcification in the ascending aorta could appear on x ray, with ST segment depression on ECG. Heart Gumma is rare. Gumma in the interventricular septum can lead to heart block.

Paroxysmal haemaglobinuria are attacks of fever, shivering and "coca-cola" coloured urine; that takes place follow exposure to cold; and are due to compliment mediated haemolyses attacks.

Congenital Syphilis

Congenital Syphilis has reduced in developed health care systems with the introduction of ante-natal screening. Despite treatment during pregnancy, 1 in 10 neonates may be affected with Syphilis. The increasing patients' unacceptability of injections during pregnancy has led some clinicians to explore alternative treatments (e.g., Azithromycin). Patients allergic to Penicillin also pose a therapeutic dilemma. There have been reports of treatment failures with both Erythromycin and Azithromycin. If the mother is treated with Macrolides, the newborn should be treated with Penicillin. Maternal desensitisation to Penicillin is possible but is care intensive and requires a committed patient; which proves difficult in patients with competing social pressures.

Transplacental transmission of Syphilis can take place at any trimester. It may lead to abortion, foetal demise and stillbirth. It may lead to maternal Polyhydraminos and foetal Hydrops. The possibility of congenital Syphilis is higher with active disease during early pregnancy; indicated by high titre of RPR/VDRL. The risk is high when Syphilis has not been treated until late in pregnancy (e.g., last trimester).

Early congenital Syphilis, in the first 2 years, may present with skin rash, Vesiculo-bullous lesions, mucous membrane lesions (leading to snuffles and/or haemorrhagic rhinitis, mucous patches), Condylomata lata and/or perioral fissures. The newborn may have generalised lymphadenopathy and hydrops. Bone manifestations include periostitis and osteochondritis. Small vessel involvement can lead to nephritis, neurological and/or occular involvement. The newborn may present with episodes of haemolysis and thrombocytopenia.

Late congenital Syphilis, after 2 years, could be characterised by stigmata (e.g., frontal bossing, short mandible, saddle-shaped deformity of the nose, sterno-clavicular thickening, high palatal arch, Mulberry molars, Hutchinson's incisors and/or Clutton's joints). Interstitial Keratitis may be the only sign that leads an ophthalmologist to suspect the diagnosis at childhood, adulthood or senior age. The child may present with paroxysmal cold haemoglopinuria, Gumma or Neuro- Syphilis.

Practical Considerations

1. In genital ulcerations a pro-active process of clinical and serological exclusion of Syphilis should be applied.
2. Genital ulcers should be considered Syphilitic in nature unless proved otherwise.
3. Antibiotics that are inactive against T pallidum should be used to treat secondary infection in a genital ulcer undergoing investigation for Syphilis. This will provide a window of opportunity for repeating the Dark Ground Microscopy tests and avoid interference with the serology tests. The accurate diagnosis of Syphilis, helps managing the patient's own condition and that of the sexual contact/s.
4. For clinical and epidemiological reasons, we consider syphilis as early, for primary, secondary and early-latent syphilis; when it is practical to follow sex contacts who are at risk of acquisition.
5. In late syphilis, late latent, the most recent sex contacts are not at risk of acquisition; but exclusion, by serology tests, would prove wise.
6. Longstanding sex partners, past partners and/or children require clinical assessment and consideration for serology tests.
7. The widespread use of antibiotics, for other medical conditions (eg. Bronchitis, otitis media, septic wounds), incidentally treat concomitant and undiagnosed syphilis; leading to Incidental Treatment; which could be full or partial. Partial treatment leads to the amelioration of clinical conditions associated with late syphilis; leading to its detection on positive serology.
8. History of blood donation and antenatal tests could be of value in areas where routine screening and testing for Syphilis are performed. The timing of a past negative test could narrow the possibilities or point to the possible interval, prior to the identification of the positive Syphilis serology tests.
9. Previous attendance and investigations for STIs could be helpful in identifying the possible time of contracting the infection. History and results of investigations (VDRL/RPR/TPHA) could be obtained from another clinic, with the patient's permission and consnt.

10. The patient's sexual history and the syphilis serology status of the partner/s could help to identify the source and stage of infection.

11. Patients who live in areas endemic with other Treponemal infections (e.g Yaws or Pinta) need careful clinical analysis of a positive Treponemal serology. The presence of leg scars could be suggestive of Yaws.

12. The clinician should consider the possibility of concomitant conditions (e.g., past Endemic Treponemal condition and superimposed infection with Syphilis). In this situation, it would be prudent to discuss the condition fully with the patient and offer treatment, as if for Syphilis.

13. Positive serology tests for Syphilis, in the absence of clinical prove or history of therapy, should be considered for treatment; as for late latent Syphilis.

Investigations

The diagnosis of Syphilis is made through a high index of clinical suspicion in certain at risk patient groups; benefiting from clinical experience and Public Health data. The recent outbreaks in the UK in "men having sex with men" and clients of certain leisure facilities (e.g., saunas) are examples. A positive serology test may be encountered following ante-natal screening, outreach care for sex workers and their clients or blood donation. Certain clinical conditions (e.g., Interstitial-Keratitis) may prompt investigations. The well informed and attentive patient may suspect the diagnosis (e.g., following the finding of a chancre). The clinician should apply a process of exclusion for patients presenting with a history of casual sexual intercourse. A full genital, general, cardiovascular and neurological examination should be tailored to the patient's own clinical history and conditions.

1) Dark- Ground Microscopy

The test is useful for penile and vulval lesions, but not suitable for oral lesions; as commensal- treponemes interfere with the certainty of diagnosis. It is less reliable for rectal and non-penile genital lesions. If chancres co-exist with secondary or congenital Syphilis, the chancre serum material could be used for Dark Ground Microscopy. Samples from Condylomata Lata and/or mucus patches could be used as well as serum aspirate from regional lymph nodes, in secondary Syphilis. Genital chancres may provide a positive test, with up to 80% sensitivity, in primary Syphilis.

The ulcer/chancre requires cleansing with a swab soaked in sterile saline. The clinician can obtain serum by gently squeezing the ulcer from side to side, collecting the serum with the edge of a cover slide, smear the sample on a slide and mount it with normal saline. A special Dark-Ground microscopy lens set is required; where the direction of light is deflected by its contact with the unstained treponemes, leading to its illumination against the Dark-Ground field. The organisms appear as a spirochaete, with a forward and backward movement and axial rotation. The organism is angulated at some 90° and have a characteristic tight spiral.

2) Serology

The serology tests are common for both Syphilis and other Endemic treponematoses. A clinical process of exclusion is required. In conflicting conditions it would be safer to treat as Syphilis.

A) Non-Specific Serology Tests, with Non Treponemal Antigens

Venereal Disease Research Laboratory (VDRL)Tests: The test is non-specific and use Cardiolipin-Antigen (Reagin) and are inexpensive. It has poor sensitivity in late Syphilis. Biological false positive results may take place with pregnancy, auto immune conditions (e.g., Lupus Erythematosous), drug reactions, acute febrile conditions (e.g., Viral Hepatitis, Infectious Mononucleosis) and vaccinations.

Quantitative tests (titres) are of value in the follow-up of treatment and identifying superimposed new infections; following a previous course of treatment. This is useful in high-risk patients (e.g men having sex with men, sex workers and their clients).

A strongly positive sample may have blocking antibodies and lead to a false negative result (Prozone phenomenon); which is likely in HIV infected individuals and require clinical attention.

Rapid plasma regain (RPR) is a modified VDRL test; which is simple, rapid and could be done in an office. Reactive results should be confirmed by another specific test.

B) Specific Serology Tests For Anti Treponemal Antibodies

1) *Treponema pallidum Haemagglutination Assay (TPHA) & Treponema pallidum Particles Aglutination Assay (TPPA):* The test could be used for either screening, confirmation or both. It gives a permanent result and is. therefore, a marker of past infection.

2) *Enzyme Immuno Assay (EIA):* Automated EIA tests are useful for mass screening and confirmation. Its early serological response can help early detection.

3) *Fluorescent Treponemal Antibody absorbed (FTA abs) tests:* are used for confirmation and early detection

4) *Specific Anti Treponemal Immunoglobulin M (IgM):* IgM provide an early serological response. It could be detected as early as the end of the second week of infection. An increasing IgM level may indicate a recent/new infection. The IgM protein size does not allow it to cross blood-placental barrier. It is, therefore, helpful in the diagnosis of congenital Syphilis. A positive syphilis specific IgM test after three month of age is an indication of a neonatal response and congenital syphilis.

3) Syphilis Polymerase Chain Reaction (PCR)

Syphilis PCR tests are performed in specialised and Public Health Reference Laboratories. The tests are time consuming and of limited availability. It is of special help for testing tissue samples, Cerebro-Spinal Fluid (CSF) and vitreous fluid. It could be used to test samples from areas where commensal Treponemes are likely to contaminate the sample (e.g., oral cavity).

4) Rapid Tests for Syphilis

The WHO is promoting the development of rapid tests for Syphilis; that are simple, do not need equipment, easy to perform outside laboratory conditions and require minimal training. A finger-prick whole blood sample is required. The tests are relevant for developing countries and outreach health care settings. They can not distinguish between active or past treated Treponemal infection, which is a disadvantage. Some 20 brands are available; with claimed test sensitivity ranging between 58-98% and specificity of 93-98%.

Investigations for Suspected Cardiovascular Syphilis

All patients diagnosed with latent Syphilis should be investigated for Tertiary disease (ie cardiovascular, neurosyphilis, ocular Syphilis …). Echo-cardiography, Ultrasonography, Computerised Tomography and/or Angiography help to make or exclude the diagnosis of for aortic incompetence and/or aortic aneurisms. The aneurismal aortic dilatation, with "eggshell" calcification, may appear on a plain chest X ray.

Investigations for Suspected Neurosyphilis

The clinical analysis of benefits versus risks, of lumbar punctures in asymptomatic late Syphilis, weighed against the procedure. The availability of effective treatments for Neurosyphilis makes the risk of lumbar puncture questionable, as the condition could be treated as for tertiary syphilis.

A negative VDRL serology test is not likely to be associated with CSF abnormalities that are compatible with Neurosyphilis. A VDRL titre of 1:32 or higher is predictive of CSF abnormalities.

CSF examination is indicated in the presence of neurological and/or ophthalmic conditions, suggestive of Syphilitic origin and/or suspected treatment failure. The CSF sample should not be contaminated with any blood; which may give a false positive result.

CSF tests indicative of neurosyphilis are: an increased white cell count, of more than $5x10^6$ /L, a high proteinof more than 0.4 gm/L, positive CSF VDRL and CSF TPPA tests.

A positive CSF lipid antigen tests (VDRL, RPR) is diagnostic of Neurosyphilis; when blood contamination is excluded. A negative CSF VDRL or RPR does not exclude Neurosyphilis; as it may be false negative in 1 in 4 neurosyphilis.

A negative CSF Treponemal Antigen test (TPHA, FTA abs) excludes Neurosyphilis, whilst a positive one is not specific and could take place in deranged blood- brain barrier (e.g., an episode of non-Syphilitic meningitis).

TPHA Index: A formula that uses CSF TPHA, CSF albumin and serum albumin; provide a reliable test for Neurosyphilis with high sensitivity and specificity. It allows for a breach in the blood brain barrier.

Investigations for Syphilis during Pregnancy

All pregnant women must be screened for Syphilis at the time of first confirmation of pregnancy. Positive cases for Syphilis benefit from early treatment; therefore, delayed screening is not justifiable. There is a case for repeated screening in high prevalence areas or at risk patients (e.g., at 28 and 32 weeks pregnancy). Penicillin G is effective during pregnancy and should be the main line of treatment. Syphilitic pregnant women who are allergic to Penicillin should be desensitised and treated with Penicillin. Non Penicillin based treatment options have reported high failure rates.

Investigations for Congenital Syphilis

The course and follow-up of infants born to Syphilitic mothers requires frequent clinical assessment and investigations, which may prove difficult to achieve in certain social circumstances (e.g., non-compliant mother, social displacement, competing interests for other children, …). Coupled with the possibility of 1 in 10 babies being affected, despite maternal treatment, some guidelines pontificate treatment of infants delivered to Syphilitic mothers; even when the mother had treatment.

Monitoring the newborn for Syphilis includes physical examination to exclude early and/or late stigmata of congenital Syphilis. Suspicious lesions may yield samples for Dark-Ground microscopy or PCR. Quantitative VDRL/RPR and TPPA tests, in both mother and baby, and Treponemal IgM EIA provide guidance for diagnosis and care. A maternal/foetal VDRL/RPR titre or TPPA titre of 4-fold or higher, with positive IgM EIA test suggests congenital Syphilis. A Negative IgM and neonatal titres less than 4-fold higher than maternal titers, with no suspicious signs of congenital Syphilis suggest that the newborn is not affected. The titres should be repeated 3-monthly and are expected to become negative at 6 months of age; as the neonate metabolises the maternal antibodies.

Negative neonatal serology with no clinical signs in the newborn indicates no congenital Syphilis and no need for further tests. Treponemal IgM EIA should be repeated at 3 months, to exclude a delayed response.

Investigations of Syphilis in HIV patients

Syphilis serological responses are unusual amongst HIV infected patients. False negative serological tests, delayed serological activity and higher than expected titres have all been reported. HIV tests should be offered to all patients who reported positive for Syphilis and be repeated after 3 months, if the first HIV result was negative. Alternative tests (e.g., Dark Field Microscopy and/or biopsy) might be helpful.

Practical Considerations

1. Screening a specific population group for Syphilis require a primary test and a confirmatory one:
   Primary Tests: EIA (preferably a test to detect both IgG and IgM), TPPA, VDRL/RPR or TPHA
   Confirmatory test are used for positive samples, and should utilizes a different Treponemal antibody test.
   Treponema pallidum Recombinant Antigen Line Immuno Assay. The test has proved useful when the standard confirmatory tests do not confirm a positive Treponemal screening test result.
2. FTA-abs should not be used as a standard confirmatory test.
3. It would be wise to take a second specimen and repeat the tests, following a positive result, to avoid clerical mistakes and/or mix-up of samples, due to the implication of a positive diagnosis on the individual, partner and relationships.
4. A quantitative VDRL/RPR baseline test, on the first day of treatment provide guidance on response to therapy.
5. VDRL or RPR titre of more than 16 and/or positive IgM test indicate an active disease and the requirement of treatment.
6. A repeat serology test (including FTA and IgM) should be used in conditions where there is a history of high risk exposure or a genital ulcer that did not yield a Dark ground field positive result. The tests should be repeated at six weeks and three months, from the point of exposure/risk.
7. VDRL/RPR and EIA/IgM are often negative in late Syphilis. Unless there is a clear history of adequate treatment, choice of antibiotic, dosage and duration, the clinician should recommend a course of treatment, for late Syphilis.

8. A high VDRL/RPR titre in late Syphilis should raise the possibility of an active condition or new re-infection.

Management of Syphilis

Treatment Principles

The efficacy of Penicillin in the treatment of Syphilis is established from case studies and over 50 years of clinical experience. There are no comparative trials to guide optimal Penicillin dose, duration and preparation. Data on non-Penicillin regimens are based on case series.

Therapeutic Regimen for adults

A) Primary Syphilis:
Benzathine Penicillin G (2.4 million units IM in a single dose), or
Procaine Penicillin (750 mg, once daily, IM for ten days), or
Doxycycline (100 mg orally twice daily for fourteen days), or
   Amoxycillin (500 mg, orally, four times daily for fourteen days) plus
   Probenecid (500 mg, orally, four times daily for fourteen days).
B) Secondary and early Latent Syphilis
Benzathine Penicillin G (2.4 million units, IM, repeated after a week), or Procaine Penicillin (750 mg, once daily, IM for fourteen days), or
   Doxycycline (100 twice daily orally for twenty one days)
C) Asymptomatic Late Syphilis:
Benzathine Penicillin (2.4 million units, weekly for three doses), or
Procaine Penicillin (750 mg, once daily, IM for seventeen days), or
Doxycycline (200 mg, orally, twice daily for twenty-eight days).
D) Cardiovascular Syphilis and Gummata are managed as asymptomatic late Syphilis.
E) Neurosyphilis:
   Procaine Penicillin (2.0 g, IM, once daily for seventeen days) plus
   Probenecid (500 mg, orally, four times daily for seventeen days), or
   Aqueous Crystalline Penicillin G (24 million units/day, continuous infusion for fourteen days), or

Doxycycline (200 mg, orally, twice daily for twenty eight days), or
Amoxycillin (2 gm, orally, three times daily for twenty eight days) plus
Probenecid (500 mg, orally, four times daily for twenty eight days).

Additional Steroid therapy is indicated, for patients with Cardio-vascular, CNS, ophthalmic or acoustic Syphilitic conditions

Clinical Practicalities

1) Probenecid is not a licensed drug in the UK.
2) Procaine Penicillin preparations are difficult to source in some countries, due to decline in its manufacturing.
3) The efficacy of Penicillin alternatives is not ideal; but may be a compromise for a patient with Penicillin Allergy; or who categorically refuses to accept injections.
4) For Cardio-vascular and Neuro-syphilis, the patient should be well informed on the lower efficacy and possibility of failed therapy for Penicillin alternatives.
5) Criteria for cure, following treatment of Syphilis, had not been established.
6) Treatment failure can occur with any regimen.
7) As with many other STIs, treatment failure is sometimes difficult to distinguish from re-infection.
8) A fourfold increase in non-Treponemal test titre, compared with the maximum titre at the time of treatment, should raise the question of re-infection versus failed treatment.
9) Failure of non-Treponemal test titres to decline fourfold within 6 months after therapy might indicate treatment failure.
10) The recommended dosage for re-treatment is Benzathine Penicillin (G 2.4 million units, IM, weekly, for three weeks).
11) It is prudent to reassess the patient's clinical condition and repeat tests, following treatment, after 6 and 12 months.
12) Syphilis with HIV infection requires more frequent evaluation (e.g., 3-monthly intervals).

Jarisch-Herxheimer reaction is a febrile illness occurring within 24 hours after treatment, with generalised symptoms, headache and myalgia. It is more common in early Syphilis. It requires general management with bed rest, hydration and antipyretics. The patient should be warned of its occurrence. During pregnancy, it may induce labour; but should not be a cause of delayed treatment.

Therapeutic Regimens for Congenital Syphilis

Aquous Crystalline Penicillin (50,000 units/kg/day, twice daily for seven days; then three times daily for three days).

Treatment of Syphilis in early pregnancy is the most effective in preventing congenital disease. Treatment within the last four weeks prior to delivery is inadequate for preventing congenital disease and treatment of the newborn should be considered. Data indicate that treatment at 28 or 32 weeks of gestation may be inadequate and evaluation and follow up of the newborn for congenital syphilis is essential.

Therapeutic Regimen for Syphilis in children

Benzathine Penicillin G (50,000 units/Kg IM up to the adult dose of 2.4 million units in a single dose).

Clinical Practicalities

1) Newborn cases considered for Syphilis treatment are defined by the history of maternal treatment, or lack of it.
2) There is a possibility of one of ten infants, born of mothers treated for Syphilis during pregnancy, to acquire the condition, despite adequate maternal treatment.
3) Syphilis in children, beyond the post-delivery period, should raise the question of Congenital versus Acquired Syphilis; where child sexual abuse should be excluded.
4) A stillborn infant, delivered after 20 weeks of pregnancy should be considered for maternal serology tests for Syphilis.

Endemic Treponematoses

Endemic Treponematoses are transmitted by direct non-venereal close contact. It affects individuals who are living, or have lived, in tropical, sub-tropical and hot countries. They may be asymptomatic or have primary, secondary and latent clinical pictures; that bear similarities to Syphilis. Improvement in hygiene, availability of antibiotics and infection control programmes has led to decline in their prevalence. Contrary to Syphilis, there is no vertical transmission, cardiovascular or neurological complications.

Yaws is caused by Treponema pertenue, and is found in warm, humid, tropical and sub-tropical areas. It is transmitted by direct skin-to-skin contact with an infectious lesion in childhood. The primary lesion is a papule that ulcerates and heals after few months by scarring. The persistent scars may aid the clinical diagnosis. The secondary lesions are skin and mucosal rash, similar to secondary Syphilis. They leave no scarring and may relapse in the first few years. They may be associated with Ostitis and periostitis and present with nocturnal pain. Gumma develop in latent stage and give skin lesions or nasal/palatal destruction and deformities.

Pinta is caused by Treponema carateum and is found in warm and semi-arid countries (e.g., South America). It is transmitted by skin-to-skin contact, usually in childhood. The infection is confined to the skin. The primary lesion is a papule, initially pink, with surrounding satellite lesions. It my change to plaque with lymphadenopathy. The secondary lesions appear pink, changing to slate-blue, then copper coloured, or lead to hypopigmented leukodermic lesions.

Endemic Syphilis (Bejel) is caused by Treponema endemicum and is found in hot, dry areas (e.g.,Saharan and Sub-Saharan Africa). It is transmitted directly by mouth-to-mouth contact during kissing or indirectly by sharing utensils. The primary lesion can lead to oral mucus patches, mucocutaneous papules and condylomata lata in children 4-10 years old. It may lead to secondary lesions that proceed to latency. Gumma develops in the skin and can lead to destruction of nose and palate.

The Human Immuno Deficiency Virus (HIV) and Acquired Immuno Deficiency Syndrome (AIDS)

History

The story of HIV started first in the USA with an epidemic of Acquired Immune-Deficiency Syndrome between young men in the early eighties. American and French researchers identified the causative virus in 1986; later called the Human Immuno Deficiency Virus (HIV). A related condition of immune deficiency was endemic in West Africa and the HIV-2 was then identified in the same year. There had been sporadic cases HIV virus detection in samples of blood or tissue, stored from as early as 1959. This suggests that the virus has existed well before the recognition of the clinical syndromes.

Prevalence

The United Nations (UN AIDS) estimates that up to 47.1 million people; of whom 20.9 million women and 3.5 million children, were living with HIV in 2006. It estimates that 6.6 million were newly infected with HIV in the same year; 660,000 of whom are children, under the age of 15. It estimates that 3.3 million AIDS deaths occurred in 2006; 500,000 of whom were children, under the age of 15. The WHO reviewed reports for 2008, indicates that while the total numbers of patients living with HIV have risen, the overall prevalence has not changed.

Two-thirds of adults and children with HIV live in Sub-Saharan Africa and one-third in Southern Africa. The proportion of women in the HIV infected population varies; between one quarter in North America, one-third in Eastern Europe and Central Asia to two-thirds in Sub-Saharan Africa. The proportion of injecting drug users in the HIV infected population varies; between two-thirds in Eastern Europe and Central Asia and one-fifth in Latin America and South East Asia. The proportion of men having sex with men in the HIV infected population is 1 in 4 in Latin America and 1 in 12-20 in Europe and Asia. The proportion of commercial sex workers in the HIV infected population is 1 in 12-20. The proportion of clients of commercial sex workers in the HIV infected population is 4 in 10 in South East Asia and 1in 10 Latin America, Asia and Europe.

HIV is now a pandemic , and one of the deadliest in human history. The WHO estimates that AIDS has killed more than 25 million people. Some 3.3 million lives were lost due to AIDS in 2005; one-third in Southern Africa. More than half a million of all deaths were children.

The USA Center for Disease Control (CDC) estimates that over a million persons were living with HIV at the end of 2003; and 35,000 new cases were diagnosed in 2006. One quarter of the HIV population are females and half are between the ages of 35 to 54. The black ethnicity accounts for half of the HIV population. Male to male sexual contact accounts for 50% of the transmission and accounts for two-thirds of all HIV infected males in the USA.

In the UK, the Health Protection Agency reported some 6,000 new cases in 2007. At the end of 2006, it estimates 73,000 HIV positive patients are living in UK; 21,600 of whom were unaware of their HIV condition.

The Virus

The HIV virus belongs to a group of viruses that uses the enzyme Reverse Transcriptase (RT or p51), to generate DNA from the host cell RNA, by a reverse transcription process (Retroviruses). The virus is composed of two identical single strands of RNA, encapsulated in a conical protein shell (Capsid). The viral RNA single strand is bound to both RT and another enzyme which enables the viral genetic material to be integrated into the host DNA (Integrase or p32). The Capsid comprise a protein (p24), that is typical of a subgroup called the Lentivirus. The Capsid is surrounded by an envelope, which is formed during budding of the virus from the host cell, and is made of viral protein and host cell membrane lipids. The envelope is two layers of Phospholipids, with transmembrane glycoprotein (gp41) and docking glycoprotein (gp120). The Glycoproteins attach the virus to the host cell, initiating infection. The Glycoprotein complex is the target of extensive investigations, research and trials for HIV vaccines.

Replication

The HIV replication cycles start with attachment of the viral Glycoprotein (gp120) to the CD4 receptors, present in mainly on helper T Lymphocytes, but also on Macrophages, Monocytes, Microglial, Dendritic, and Langerhans cells. Structural changes take place in the Glycoprotein (gp41) leading to the fusion of both viral and host cell membranes; followed by the infusion of the viral material into the host cell. Viral RNA, Reverse Transcriptase enzyme (p51), Integrase enzyme (p32), Matrix (p17) and Nucleocapsid interact with various host proteins to produce double DNA strand of HIV pre-integration complex. Integrase enzyme integrates the viral DNA with the host cell chromosomes. A pro virus is transcribed and eventually the HIV viral material (Virion) is released from the host cell by a budding process, during which it acquires a membrane formed of viral protein and host cell lipids. The process can produce 100 million to 10 billion viral particles per day.

HIV I is divided into Main group (M), with sub-types (A-I), some with uncertain classification (U)). It is the most common and have a worldwide distribution. Outlier group (O) and New group (N) are identified in Africa. Sub-type B is mainly found in homosexual males and IV drug users and is predominant in Europe, America, Australia and the Far East. Sub-type E replicates readily in Langerhans'cells, which are found in male and female genital tracts, but not in the rectum; hence more common in heterosexuals. HIV1 is more virulent, mutates rapidly and leads to progressive clinical condition, than HIV2.

HIV 2 is divided into groups (A-G), predominant in West Africa, less virulent and leads to less vertical transmission than HIV 1.

Practical Considerations

1. Population movements, travel and immigration, will eventually blur the boundaries for the geographical distribution of HIV groups/sub-types.

2. Mutations should be considered in testing strategies. Tests should cover both HIV I and II with their groups and sub-types.
3. The continuous mutation of HIV groups and sub-types may reflect on the efficacy of treatment.
4. HIV vaccine trials face practical difficulties of providing cross protection to HIV groups, sub-types and new mutants.

Transmission

HIV transmission is mainly through intimate contact with body fluids. Genital fluids, semen in males and lower genital tract and menstrual secretions in females, provide a vehicle for viral transmission. The virus is attached to sperms or included in white cells. The viral load in the index patient and the breach of integrity of muocous membranes and skin surfaces of the recepient affect infectivity. Genital ulcerative disease (e.g., caused by Herpes Genitalis, Syphilis and/or Lymphogranuloma), promotes the possibility of transmission. Infectivity is also affected by the route of sexual intercourse. A single act of sexual intercourse has an estimated possibility of transmission of 1-2/1000 for receptive vaginal sex, 3-9/10,000 for insertive vaginal sex, 1-30/1,000 for receptive anal and 4/10,000 for insertive anal sex. The possibility of receptive oral sex is estimated at 4/10,000. There are no data on transmission via insertive oral sex.

The possibility of HIV transmission from sharing syringes/needles between drug users is estimated as 7/1,000 acts of single exposure. The use of contaminated surgical/medical equipment is thought to be a high route of transmission in areas of low health care resources. The highest possibility of transmission comes with infected blood transfusion, reaching 100%.

Data on occupational needle-stick injuries arc limited but suggestive of a chance of 3/1,000. Accidental inoculation of infected fluids into mucus membranes (e.g., conjunctival sac) carries a chance of 1/1,000.

The prevalence of HIV positivity in a background population influences the possibility of transmission in conditions, when the HIV status of the source is unknown (e.g., casual sexual intercourse, sexual assault). The physician and recipient patient need this information to make an informed decision and consent regarding the initiation of post-exposure prophylaxis (PEP).

In occupational exposure (e.g., needle-stick injury) it may be possible to obtain the Index patient's consent to volunteer a blood sample for HIV testing. A negative test result will avoid unnecessary therapy (PEP), for the injured person.

HIV test ordered on a blood sample previously taken from the Index patient, without his approval, could constitute infringement of civil liberties. The legal implications for each country or State should be carefully considered.

HIV Disease Progression

The progression of HIV disease, and its culmination into AIDS, varies according to host and viral factors. Advanced patient's age, moribund psychological status, females, poor physical and/or nutritional status lead to more progression in HIV disease. Concurrent infections (e.g., tuberculosis, malaria and cytomegalovirus) progress the disease faster. Individuals with certain Human Leucocyte Antigen (HLA) progress more slowly. Certain genetic characteristics make some individuals almost resistant to HIV infection.

The changes in viral phenotypic and genotypic characteristics and continuous process of mutations, promotes viral resistance to drugs and consequently disease progression. The use of suboptimal drug dosages and/or interruptions in the course of therapy, either due to lack of medications, suboptimal dosages or ineffective products (e.g., counterfeit drugs) can promote viral resistance and disease progression.

The continuous and progressive destruction of the host immune system, eventually allow for the unopposed opportunistic organisms to cause infections and malignancies to progress to AIDS defining conditions. If left untreated, the average interval between HIV infections and progression to AIDS is 10 years.

Primary HIV Infection (PHI) defines the period between acquisition and the host establishing an immune balance with the virus. It takes few weeks to months. It is associated with a spike of viraemia and a depression in the immune status, reflecting on a decline in the CD4 count.

Acute Retroviral Syndrome (ARS) & Acute Sero Conversion Illness define the development of HIV specific antibodies. It is associated with non specific symptoms; hence a wide range of reporting, varying between 30-90%. The syndrome is mostly reported in adults and with HIV I. The identification of the syndrome relies on the physician's index of clinical suspicion and the awareness of the suspecting patient. The non-specificity of the syndrome and/its mildness, can make it unrecognisable. The symptoms correspond to peaks of viraemia, usually 2-6 weeks after infection. There is usually pyrexia, lymphadenopathy, pharyngitis and /or skin rash. The patient may develop Infectious Mononucleosis (IM) like illness (i.e., pyrexia, pharyngitis, lymphadenopathy, arthralgia and /or myalgia). Unlike IM, the tonsils are spared in ARS. Due to immune suppression, the patient may develop oral-pharyngeal candidiasis or Pneumocystis jirovecii (carinii) pneumonia. There may be neurological effects (e.g., meningitis, encephalitis, myelopathy and/or peripheral neuropathy). The intensity and duration of the sero-conversion illness could be an indication of the future rate of HIV disease progression. Differential Diagnosis of ARS include: Infectious Mononucleosis, Viral Hepatitis, Primary/Secondary Syphilis, drug reactions, Cytomegalovirus infections, Toxoplasmosis and/or bacterial pharyngitis.

The Immune Response

The cellular immune response to HIV infection develops early and influences its natural history. The initial high levels of viraemia result from active viral replication. It is associated with viral dissemination and replication in lymphoid tissue. There is an initial stage of Lymphopenia, suppression of both CD4 and CD8; followed by a surge in CD8, leading to reversion of CD4-CD8 ratio to less than 1. At the end of this stage, a higher viral load is could be suggestive of increased risk of the future rate disease progression.

The antibody response to HIV infection may take up to three months; usually 10-21 days. Antibodies to p24 develop first but then decline and may disappear in later stage. Antibodies to gp120 and gp41 develop later but persist for life. A poor antibody response suggests disease progression and poor prognosis.

The physician's recognition of the primary infection and sero conversion stages can help to identify the most likely sexual partners; for contact tracing, investigations and care. This stage is associated with high viral levels and sexual intercourse carry higher risk of infection. There is no evidence of long-term benefits for the early initiation of treatment during the primary/sero conversion stage. Theoretically, early anti retroviral treatment may provide some protection to the host, by preserving immunity and reducing cell infectivity. The drawbacks are the possibilities of increasing drug toxicity and resistance, due to prolonged treatment. and cost implications.

HIV Natural History

Untreated HIV infection leads to progressive decline in the immune system. The progression varies between individuals, depending on the patient's own resistance and viral virulence. Eventually, the patient succumbs to opportunistic infections and malignancies; which defines the Acquired Immuno Deficiency Syndrome (AIDS). The average time between HIV infection and AIDS is 10 years, in untreated patients. Some patients may progress to AIDS, within two years of HIV acquisition.

The primary HIV infection is associated with body-wide dissemination of the virus, very high Viral Load (VL) and decline in CD4 cells. The initial CD4 decline is followed by partial reversion. The initial viraemia and high VL, declines later; and may be undetectable in rare cases. The patient may continue to be asymptomatic for several years; except from Generalised Lymphadenopathy and/or dermatological changes (e.g., Seborrhoeic Dermatitis and Psoriasis). At lower CD4 count (200-500 cells/μL) the patient becomes vulnerable to Community Acquired Pneumonias, Mycobacterium tuberculosis, recurrent Herpes simplex and/or Varicella zoster infections. The patient may present with intermittent pyrexia, diarrhoea and/or weight loss. In the advanced stage (CD4 count 50-200 cells/μL), the patient is vulnerable to, Pneumocystis jirovecii pneumonia, Karposi's Sarcoma, Lymphomas and Mycobacterium avium Complex (MAC). At the late stage, marked by CD4 count of less than 50 cells/μL and high VL, severe immune deficiency may lead to Cytomegalovirus (CMV) retinitis and/or disseminated MAC. Wasting disease, progressive dementia and neurological manifestations precede the eventual demise.

The introduction of Highly Active Anti-Retroviral Therapy (HARRT) has modified the pattern of the disease and associated conditions. In areas where the therapy is available, patients are leading close to normal life. Patients' longevity and well-being are within normal.There remains the painful fact that most HIV patients have no access to treatment, due to under-developed healthcare resources. There are patients who are afraid of the diagnosis, unsuspecting and/or unaware of their HIV condition. These patients may present with full-blown HIV related clinical syndromes.

HIV Related Respiratory Conditions

Pneumocystis jiroveci (carinii) pneumonia (PCP)

The organism was classified initially as protozoan, but later recognised as yeast. Before the introduction of effective suppressive HIV therapy, PCP was an AIDS indicator in two thirds of patients, when their CD count falls below 200 cells/µL. PCP is caused by new infection; contrary to what was previously thought to be reactivation of the latent organisms.

Symptoms and Signs

The patient presents early with a history of increasing dyspnoea and dry cough, of several weeks' duration; with constitutional symptoms and tiredness. At a later stage, there is dyspnoea at rest. Trans-cutaneous oxygen measurement (Oximetry) provides a valuable bedside test. It may be possible to demonstrate reduced oxygen saturation at rest. Otherwise, a reduction by 5% following exercise is suggestive of PCP. Pneumothorax may be the first clinical presentation.

Investigation

The interstitial nature of the condition may require high resolution Computerised Tomography (CT) scan which shows ground glass appearance in the lower lung fields. The patient's clinical condition is usually out of proportion of chest x-ray signs, which could be minimal. In severe cases, the x-ray shows basal and peri-hilar interstitial consolidation. When pentamidine prophylaxis was in wider use, upper lobe lung lesions and extra pulmonary effects of the disease were noted, as pentamidine has no systemic role in prophylaxis. The demonstration of Pneumocystis jiroveci cysts in sputum is diagnostic. Sputum induction with saline and nebuliser may produce a useful sample. Obtaining a productive sputum sample may prove difficult in patients with deranged lung functions. Bronchoscopy and lavage, for microbiological samples, or biopsy, for histological examination, will confirm the diagnosis. Staining the sample with Fluoroscene linked monoclonal antibodies, increase the diagnostic accuracy.

Management

Co-trimoxazole (120 mg/Kg) daily for 21 days, in 4 divided dosages, is the first line management. It should be initiated first and prior to HAART; to avoid synergistic toxicities. Hypersensitivity reactions are common and may be expressed in skin, haematology and/or hepatic impairments. Folinic acid is of value where there is bone marrow impairment. Alternative therapies are required in cases of hypersensitivity and include: Clindamycin (600 mg four times daily), Trimetrexate (45 mg/m^2/day IV with Folinic acid), Dapsone (100 mg/day), Trimethoprim (5 mg/kg four hourly), Atovaquone (750 mg three times daily).

The Oxygen supplement is based upon the level of respiratory impairment. Steroid therapy is required if the arterial oxygen pressure is low (less than 9.3 kPa) or there is a reduction of 20% from the basal oxygen saturation, measured on oximetry. Steroid treatment reduces the risk of respiratory failure and mortality, but increases the risk of activation of herpes simplex viral conditions and superimposed candidal infections. Prednisolone, with a starting dose of 40 mg twice daily, is maintained for 5 days, reduced gradually to 40 mg/day for another 5 days, then 20 mg/day for 10 days. Progressive respiratory failure may need intensive care measures, intubation and ventilation with constant positive airway pressure.

The introduction of HAART is leading clinicians to withdraw secondary PCP prophylaxis following stabilisation of HIV therapy, suppression of viral load and sustained increase in the CD4 count, to more than 200 cells/µL (e.g., after 6 months).

PCP is preventable by primary prophylaxis. Co-trimoxazole (960 mg orally three times weekly) is the first line. In case of drug reactions, desensitization by gradually increasing dosages is possible. Atovaquone (750 mg orally three times weekly), or Dapsone (50-100 mg daily) are alternative options.

Bacterial Pneumonia

Bacterial Pneumonia was a direct cause of high morbidity in HIV patients before the introduction of HAART. The most common pathogens are Streptococcus pneumonia, Haemophilus influenza and Staphylococcus aureus.

The clinical presentation is one of productive cough, with purulent sputum, of a few days' duration, with focal lung abnormalities on clinical assessment. The radiographic investigations would show focal lesions; possibly diffuse in advanced and late cases, that is usually segmental, lobar and unilateral. The x-ray pattern is of alveolar; rather than the granular/ reticular appearance of PCP interstitial disease. There may be pleural effusion. Staph aureus and Pseudomonas aeruginosa infections are more significant in advanced immunodeficiency. The clinician should be aware of the possibility of concomitant and superimposed infections and the atypical presentation in the severely immunocompromised.

General measures to correct for hypoxia, hypotension, dehydration and volume depletion should be instituted first. Samples for microbiological investigations, sputum and blood for cultures and antibiotic susceptibility tests and serology for atypical pneumonia should be obtained before the initiation of antibiotic therapy. Liaison with the microbiologists should help therapeutic choice, according to the concurrent prevailing trends. Intravenous Cefuroxime (1.5 g 3 times daily)or Amoxycillin (1 g three times daily) plus a Macrolide (e.g., Clarithromycin, 5 mg twice daily), should be initiated until microbiological culture and sensitivity tests dictate later regimens. There is a case for intravenous immunoglobulin therapy and prophylactic antibiotics in recurrent pneumonia, in patients with lower immunity. Institutionalised patients and the elderly are more prone to Legionella, which could be tested for by specific urine antigen.

Clinical Practicalities

1. Advancing HIV disease can lead to reduction in lung function without superimposed pulmonary infections.
2. Smoking has an adverse effect on pulmonary functions, lung defences and exaggerates the HIV-related respiratory conditions.
3. The physician can initiate therapy on clinical assessment and prior to microbiological results.

Tuberculosis (TB)

The prevalence of TB has been increasing in western societies in recent years and should be proactively excluded in HIV positive patients with pulmonary conditions. In Africa, two thirds of patients with extra pulmonary TB have HIV infection and patients presenting with TB should have HIV excluded. Most cases of TB in HIV patients are due to reactivation of past latent infection.TB has an immunosuppressive effect ; which adds to that of the HIV infection.

The clinician should adopt a high index of clinical suspicion of Tuberculosis, at any stage of the HIV disease. The patient may present with classical symptoms of cough, night fever and sweats, pleuritic pain, weight loss and haemoptysis. In advanced HIV disease, reduced immunity and lower CD4 counts, the presentation is atypical and may mimic community acquired pneumonia. Patients at low CD4 count are at risk of primary infection with TB and dissemination in extra pulmonary disease.

Investigations

The typical radiological signs of Tuberculosis are observed in patients with better immune function. In the immuno-compromised, the radiological pattern may mimic other infections. The identification of acid-fast bacilli on microscopy or culture is diagnostic; but a negative test does not exclude the diagnosis of TB, as the sputum smear positivity in HIV patients is low. Sputum induction, or bronchoscopy guided alveolar lavage, should be considered in patients unable to produce sputum. Culture tests are central to the identification of the Mycobacterium, confirmation of clinical diagnosis and drug susceptibility testing.

PCR tests and gene probes for Tuberculosis are available; but a negative result does not exclude the diagnosis. PCR tests are of value in the diagnosis of M tuberculosis from others (e.g., avium). The definitive diagnosis of M avium or M tuberculosis poses a challenge to the physician, due to the need of change in drug therapy. The drug susceptibility tests can take some 3 weeks and require the identification of the isolate first. Standard assays are performed and Rifampicin resistance could be detected by gene probes and molecular technology.

Management

Empirical Anti-Tuberculosis therapy should be initiated on the grounds of strong clinical suspicion. Clinical response is good guidance, which may dictate the continuation of anti-Tuberculosis therapy, in the absence of positive culture tests. Drug interactions, between anti-Tuberculosis and anti-HIV therapies, are significant; due to enzyme inducing and inhibiting properties of many of these therapeutics. If HAART is possible to withhold, in case of CD4 count above 100/μL, it would be wise to delay its start; until the anti-TB medications are reduced to dual therapy. Patients presenting with a CD4 count below 100/μL have a significant risk of opportunistic infections; if HAART is withheld.

HIV Related Gastro-Intestinal Conditions

Oral and Pharyngeal Conditions

Oral disease is very common in HIV patients and may be the first presentation to raise suspicion and lead to the diagnosis. There are usually signs of immuno-compromise; therefore oral disease is encountered at a later stage in patients not receiving anti-retroviral therapy.

Oral Hairy Leukoplakia (OHL) are caused by Epstein-Barr virus (EBV). The lesions are white, vary in size and adhere to the underlying mucosa, which differentiates it from oral candidiasis. They are located on the lateral aspect of the tongue and usually asymptomatic. Some patients may complain of pain or change of taste. OHL is more common in adult males who smoke; but may affect any other group. It is a sign of immuno compromise and is not unique to HIV. OHL is not pre-malignant but an indicator of progression to AIDS. The condition regresses with improvement in the patient's immune status under HAART.

Oral Candidiasis is the most common HIV related opportunistic infection; affecting most of the patient at some stage of their disease. It is a sign of immuno-compromise; therefore more common at later stage with low CD4 counts. It may be part of the sero- conversion syndrome. Candida albicans is usually implicated; but C glabrata and C tropicalis are also isolated. An overgrowth of the candidal hyphae, inflammatory and desquamated cells take the shape of a pseudo-membrane. The membrane appears as a white plaque that is removable, leaving an area of erythema, punctation and bleeding. Rarely, it is easy to remove with no underlying effects. The lesion may appear as erythematous patches, ulcers or fissures. The patient may present with change in taste, mouth soreness, burning and/ or white patches. The clinical appearance is diagnostic. Microscopic examination of a Gram- stained smear may demonstrate the hyphae. Culture is useful in identifying antifungal responsiveness. Treatment regimens include Fluconazole (orally, 50-100mg daily) or Itraconazole (orally, 100-200mg once daily), all for 1-2 weeks and guided by clinical response. Oral anti-fungals are used only in mild cases. Nystatin (100,000 – 500,000 units four times daily) as suspension or pastilles or Miconazole (5-10mL) oral gel applied to the lesion should be guided by clinical response and continued up to 2 days after recovery. Prophylactic therapy is useful in the severely immuno-compromised patient (e.g., Fluconazole 50mg, orally, once daily); but there is a risk of developing fungal resistance. Differential diagnosis includes hairy Leukoplakia, Lichen Planus, Syphilitic mucous patches, Intraepithelial Neoplasia and Basal Cell Carcinoma.

Periodental Disease, Gingivitis, Linear Gingival Erythema, Necrotizing Ulcerative Peri-odontitis, Necrotizing Stomatitis and dental abscesses are all common with HIV infection. Mild conditions of gingival erythema and oedema, respond to oral hygiene, Chlorhexidine mouth wash and Metronidazole treatment. Severe conditions progress to Necrotizing Periodontitis or Stomatitis; leading to destruction of periodontal tissue and bone or necrosis of localised areas of the mouth. The progress is rapid and the early expertise of oral specialists should be thought in the management. The condition may require debridement of the necrotic tissue and bone.

Herpes Simplex Viral (HSV) lesions are prevalnt and increasing; especially in homosexual males. The primary episode may present as vesicles, ulcerations or healing lesions. It affects any part of the mouth. There could be other oro-pharyngeal lesions that could be identified on endoscopy. There is no associated viraemia. The virus lies dormant in the trigeminal ganglia, during the latent stage. The active attacks are usually more severe, frequent and prolonged in the immuno-compromised HIV patient. Recurrent episodes affect the mucocutaneous junction. Some patients may experience a prodroma of pain or tingling sensation, prior to the active lesion.

Cytomegalovirus (CMV) serum positivity in HIV patients is high and increases with advancing age, especially in homosexual males. The CMV oral lesions are solitary necrotic ulcers with red margin. They could be difficult to differentiate from Herpes Simplex or Zoster ulcers lesions. The significance of CMV diagnosis is that systemic and disseminated disease affects patients with a very low CD4 count (< 50 cells/µL) and carries serious consequences (e.g., CMV retinitis). The virus lie dormant in the trigeminal nerve and its activation leads into skin lesions that may take weeks to recover. The oral lesions appear as vesicles followed by painful ulcers.

Oral warts are more common in HIV patients and are not influenced by the stage of the disease. Management would involve surgical removal, cryotherapy or laser. Local anaesthesia could be used.

HIV associated oral ulcerations are common and vary in size. Small ulcers of 2mm appear in groups in the mouth and/or soft palate. "Aphthous Minor" are medium-sized, 1cm in diameter, superficial, circumscribed and solitary. "Aphthous Major" are larger ulcers, of more than 2cm in diameter, found in the posterior mouth, pharynx or naso-pharynx. They are painful lesions that persist for weeks. The treatment is challenging and the choice is judged by the patient's other circumstances. Topical steroids are effective with small and medium-sized lesions (e.g.,Colbetasol). Systemic steroids (Prednisolone 50mg, orally, daily for

10 days) are required when topical steroids are ineffective or inapplicable. Thalidomide (200mg/day) proved effective but restrictions on pregnancies must apply. The differential diagnosis includes Herpes simplex, Herpes zoster and Cytomegalovirus ulcerations, Syphilitic or myco-bacterial lesions, Necrotizing Stomatitis and Behcet's disease.

Oral Kabosi's Sarcoma is an AIDS defining condition; less encountered in patients on HAART. The lesions may range from macule, papule, nodule, to a large mass. The latter may ulcerate and be complicated with secondary infections.

Oesophageal disease usually presents as Dysphagia. Candidal Oesophagitis is the most common cause and could be diagnosed and treated on empirical basis. Other aetiology of Dysphagia includes conditions affecting the immune compromised patient; like Herpes Simplex, Cytomegalovirus, Kabosi's Sarcoma and/or Lymphomas, or non-HIV related conditions (e.g., Reflux Oesophagitis). Endoscopy and multiple biopsies are essential to identify, or exclude, concurrent conditions. Fluconazole or Itraconazole (200mg, orally, once daily, for 1-2 weeks) is usually effective. Resistant Candidiasis is rare but would benefit from the improved Bio-availability of Itraconazole suspension (200mg, orally, twice daily, for 2 weeks). Liposomal Amphotericin B is valuable in refractory conditions.

HIV Related Kaposi's Sarcoma (KS)

Kaposi's Sarcoma is the most common HIV associated malignancy. It is caused by the Human Herpes Virus (HHV-8). Saliva and oral contacts play a significant role in transmission. HHV-8 is rarely detected in semen, which casts doubt on the role of sexual intercourse in transmission. It may be transmitted by organ transplant or mother-to-child contact. The condition affects mostly homosexual males; females are rarely affected and possibly from a bisexual male. KS is a definitive diagnosis for AIDS. Before HAART, it identified one in five 5 patients; and half of the AIDS patients had evidence of KS. Its incidence is decreasing following the introduction of HAART. Patients on immuno-suppressant therapy may also develop KS; which resolves after stopping the drugs.

KS skin lesions may affect any part of the body. Facial involvement causes patient anxiety, as the KS lesions may reveal the patient's HIV condition. Patienta are concerned that gay communities' awareness of HIV associated conditions may identify the status of a patient with KS skin lesions. The lesion may range from several millimetres to centimeters. It presents as macule, plaque or a nodule. The colour is usually deep purple to dark brown, depending on the patient's own skin tan. It may lead to ulcerations, bleeding and/or secondary infection. Feet and sole lesions can cause incapacitating pain. KS bleeding could be alarming to the patient and physician (e.g., Haemoptysis from lung lesions; or lower gastrointestinal bleeding). Visual lesions may not be symptomatic but discovered accidentally, during the course of investigations. Lung lesions may present with cough, dyspnoea, haemoptysis; or found incidentally on a chest X-ray. The radiological appearance may take the form of nodules, areas of infiltrations or lymphadenopathy. KS lesions may affect any organ or lymph nodes. Direct infiltration to lymphatics leads of Lymphoedema.

The diagnosis of KS relys upon the clinical appearance and could be confirmed by biopsy. The prognosis depends on the progress and spread of KS, stage of HIV, CD4 count and Viral Load, response to HAART and/or concurrent opportunistic infections. The prognosis is poor with systemic KS disease.

Patients are usually concerned with the cosmetic appearance and disfiguring effect of KS, especially on exposed parts (e.g., face and hands). Camouflage cosmetic interventions are non invasive but successful in bringing a skin tone similar to that of the adjacent areas. Cryotherapy is an option and lead to lesion shrinkage; but may leave hyper-pigmented areas. Topical radiotherapy is effective and useful for painful lesions (eg. Feet) and accessible space occupying lesion (eg. Oro-pharynx or eye socket). Intralesional injection of cytotoxic materials (Vincristine) or alpha interferon could be used for muco-cutaneous KS. Alpha interferon had good results with early skin KS; but should be used in patients with no history of opportunistic infections and who have a higher CD4 count. The side-effects are remarkable and the drug should be weighed against other topical alternatives.

Liposomal chemotherapy, given systemically, has a direct effect on vascular KS lesions. It has satisfactory outcomes in extensive skin/visceral lesions. It could be used in patients with lower CD4 counts but may produce neutropenia.

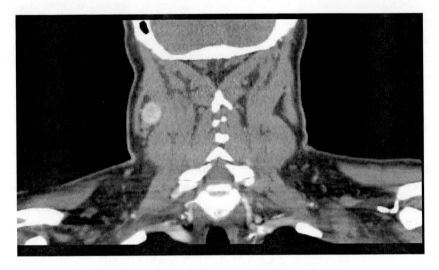

Figure 1. CT scane showing Pharyngeal KS

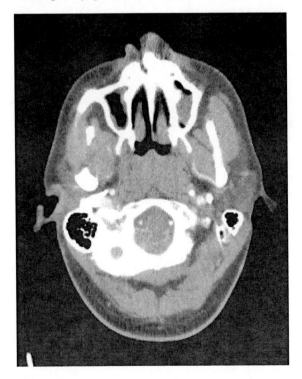

Figure 2. CT scane showing Pharyngeal KS

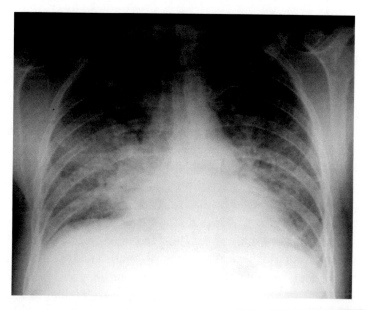

Figure 3. Chest X-ray showing PCP changes

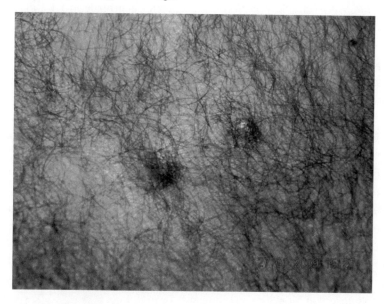

Figure 4. Skin Kaposi Sarcoma

HIV Related Skin Conditions

Dermatological disorders associated with immune-deficiency have atypical clinical picture and poor response to therapy in the untreated HIV patient. HAART leads to spontaneous improvement in HIV related skin diseases; and sometimes, complete resolution.

Seborrhoeic Dermatitis(SD) is a common occurrence in HIV patients. It affects most of the patients, with increasing frequency at later stages with CD4 decline. Mitigating factors are a combination of infection with Pityrosporum species, patient genetic factors and increased sebum. The patient may present early with butterfly erythematous rash, which could be confused with Rosacea. The associated itching, greasy skin and scales are characteristic of SD. It affects the scalp. In severe cases, it affect the chest and intertriginous areas. Mild cases respond to combination of topical Anti-fungals and steroids (e.g., Clotrimazole and Hydrocortisone). Selenium Sulphide and tar-containing shampoos are needed for scalp lesions. Systemic anti-fungals (e.g., Itraconazole) may be required for severe conditions.

Eczema, with variable severity, is a frequent occurrence in HIV disease and increases with the CD4 decline. Dry skin and itching is common presentation and responds well to emollients. Excessive scratching can lead to Lichenification and severe eczematous changes; and may require topical steroids.

Cutaneous Candidiasis is common with HIV infection. It can take the form of acute or chronic paronychia, intertrigo or tinea unguium. The causative organism is the Candida Species. Most require systemic anti-fungals. Topical preparations give satisfactory results in acute paronychia and intertrigo, other conditions require systemic anti-fungals.

Tinea pedis, cruris, corporis, capitis, faciale are very common in HIV infection. Tinea pedis should proactively be treated and it responds well at the early stage to topical anti-fungals. The macerated skin may lead to secondary infections and cellulites. Other Tinea conditions require systemic anti-fungals (e.g., Fluconozole, 30mg daily).

Skin Cryptococcosis and Histoplasmosis could be part of systemic infections; and the management of the systemic disease takes priority. The conditions are usually diagnosed on biopsy of a skin papule or nodule.

Norwegian Scabies may occur in advanced HIV disease. The early treatment of suspected and/or diagnosed scabies circumvent progression. It is highly infectious and barrier nursing is required. Treatment is systemic with either Ivermectin 200 μg/kg in a single dose, in addition to topical treatment.

Acute Retroviral Syndrome patients present with infectious mononucleosis like rash at the stage of acute sero conversion. The rash is typically macular or maculo-papular, non-itchy and symmetrical; rarely vesiclular or pustular. Aphthous ulcerations, oral, pharyngeal and/or genital, should raise clinical suspicion of sero conversion.

Herpes simplex virus (HSV) skin lesions, in advanced HIV disease, become atypical. The ulcers are larger, chronic and painful. Peri-oral, genital and perianal lesions are encountered. There is a risk of auto-inoculation. Diagnosis by Polymerase Chain Reaction (PCR) testing of skin swabs give rapid and satisfactory answers, when available. Viral culture and confirmation with immuno-fluorescent tests (IF) are time-consuming. Treatment should be initiated on empirical basis, when PCR culture and IF are not available, the finding of the multi-nucleate giant epithelial cells on histological samples can support the diagnosis.

Varicella zoster virus (VZV) in adults previously exposed to VZV, develop Herpes Zoster; affecting multiple dermatomes; with thoracic and trigeminal nerve distribution. The patient has a prodromal attack of tingling and burning, followed by vesicles. In advanced HIV disease, the condition is aggressive; causing painful haemorrhagic and necrotic lesions, persist for weeks, heal with scarring, recurrent and disseminate widely. Rarely hyperkeratotic lesions develop and are Acyclovir resistant. The diagnosis is based on the clinical picture. Biopsy makes the diagnosis in atypical ulceration, chronic and hyperkeratotic lesions. Treatment with intravenous Acyclovir (10mg/kg body weight, three times daily) is indicated for disseminated VZV, low CD4 (below 200 cells/µL) and/or ophthalmic involvement. This is followed with oral Acyclovir, at the higher dosage (800mg five times daily), which should start with clinical improvement. The improved bioavailability of Famciclovir (500mg three times daily) and Valacilovir (1gm three times daily) provide a therapeutic alternative. The course of therapy is 7-10 days and should be guided by clinical improvement.

Molluscum Contagiosum may mark an advanced HIV disease; with widespread lesions reaching 1cm in size and affecting face and trunk. Cryotherapy, curetage and topical Podophyllotoxin provide a choice of therapy that could be guided by the lesion site and patient's preference.

Warts and Human Papilloma Virus infections may affect the immuno-compromised HIV patient with recurrent and widespread lesions. The treatment principles are the same as for non-HIV patients.

Bacterial skin infections increase with the degree of immuno-suppression. Infection with Staphylococcus aureus may present as Folliculitis in hirsute areas,

Hidradenitis-like plaques, Bullous Impetigo and/or Erythema and ulceration. The conditions usually respond to anti-staphylococcal antibiotics (e.g., Flucloxacillin 500mg, four times daily, for seven days). A longer course is required for deeper infections and abscesses should be drained.

Bacillary angiomatosis cause cutaneous and sub-cutaneous angiogenic lesions that are difficult to differentiate from Kaposi's Sarcoma. The lesions are hyperpigmented papules, nodules or plaques that may be solitary, multiple and widespread and bleed easily. Bacteraemia could be associated with Pyrexia. Organ dissemination may involve the liver, spleen, bone and/or lymph nodes. Diagnosis is achieved with histology, special staining and electron microscopy.

HIV Associated Malignancies

Hodgkin's Disease is not an AIDs defining condition. It is usually associated with low CD4 counts (below 300 cells/μL); in association with Epstein Barr virus (EBV). The patient presents with pyrexia, anaemia and lymphadenopathy and the diagnosis is made on histology for lymph node and/or bone marrow samples. Early stages are treated with radiotherapy and combination of cytotoxics and steroids for later stage disease.

Non-Hodgkin's Lymphoma (NHL) accounts for 1 in 10 cases of untreated AIDS patients; with improving survival since the introduction of HAART. The patient presents with lymphadenopathy, fever, weight loss and/or indications of organ involvement (e.g., gastrointestinal tract or central nervous system and/or bone marrow). Evidence of EBV is found in most CNS cases; and in variable proportions of others. The diagnosis is made by histology on a biopsy from the suspected lesion. Bone marrow biopsy and whole body computerised tomography (CT) and MRI scan are required for staging. Treatment benefits from a multidisciplinary team management and an oncologist with expertise in the management of HIV associated NHL. Treatment regimens include combination of cytotoxic drugs and steroids. The course of therapy may require correction of neutropenia and PCP prophylaxis. Monoclonal antibody (e.g., Rituximab) could be used either in combination with chemotherapy or in resistant cases.

Primary Effusion Lymphoma is lymphoma of serous cavity membranes and is associated with HHV 8. It leads to ascites, pleural and/or pericardial effusions and carries a poor prognosis.

Primary Central Nervous System Lymphoma is EBV induced and is encountered at lower CD4 counts, of below 50 cells/μL. The diagnosis is aided with the identification of lymphoma cells or positive PCR for EBV in a cerebro-spinal fluid sample. It shares clinical similarities with Toxoplasmosis. Serology tests for Toxoplasmosis aids in the differential diagnosis. The introduction of HAART has improved survival; otherwise, radiotherapy and combination chemotherapy are used, but with poor prognosis.

Invasive Cervical Cancer is an AIDS defining condition. There is evidence of increased cervical dysplasia with immuno-suppression. There is no evidence of increased incidence of cervical cancer in HIV patients that is not accountable for by co-factors. The management of abnormal cervical cytology should follow general guidance, with more attention to early pro-active intervention and closer follow-up. Cervical cytology should be offered on a yearly basis and repeated 6-monthly for patients who have had intraepithelial Neoplasia. Higher grade CIN (CIN II and III) benefits from an excision biopsy, as a therapeutic and diagnostic methods; to ascertain that there is no invasion. The introduction of HPV Typing, with the identification of oncogenic HPV types can add a clinical value in the identification and early follow-up of patients at high risk of progressive lesions.

Anal Intraepithelial Neoplasia and *anal cancer* are 80-fold higher in homosexual males than controls. There is a case for routine anal cytology, to detect dyskaryotic cellular changes early; which should consequently be assessed with anoscopy; and biopsy of suspected lesions. Anal/Peri-anal Intraepithelial Neoplasia would benefit from excision biopsy, to exclude invasion, which would require more extensive treatment.

Lung cancer is eight times more common in HIV infected individuals than controls. The improved survival with HAART has contributed to a rise in incidence. The patient presents with cough, haemoptysis and/or chest pain; when the condition is suspected on chest x-ray. The clinician needs to have a high degree of clinical suspicion, to make an early diagnosis and timely treatment; otherwise, the prognosis is poor.

HIV related CNS conditions

HIV readily crosses the blood brain barrier, affecting microglial cells and microphages. At seroconversion, variable degrees of presentation may range from meningitis, encephalitis, myelopathy to neuropathy, including cranial nerve syndromes. At severe immuno-defeciency, there is a risk of CNS opportunistic infections and/or malignancies.

HIV associated Dementia affect the later disease stage; with degeneration of the subcortical grey matter.It presents with cognetive, psychiatric and/or personality disorders; but the initiation of HAART could reverse some of the deterioration. The patient and carers need support in addition to pharmaco-therapy.

Cerebral toxoplasmosis, caused by Toxoplasma gondii, was once a common aetiology of mass accupying lesions. The introduction of PCP prophylaxis reduced its incidence. An enhancement aroud the lesion may chracterise the CT/MRI picture. Toxoplasma serology is positive in most cases. Differential diagnosis include lymphoma, TB and cryptococcal lesions.

Cryptococcal meningitis, caused by Cryptococcous neoformans, could be covert in subacute disease, presenting with headach and/or pyrexia. It requires clinical awareness and the detection of Cryptococcal antigen in serum or CSF confirm the diagnosis. HIV meningitis may be part of seroconversion.

Progressive Multifocal Leukoencephalopathy (PML) is a demylinated disease affecting one in twelve late stage patients, in subacute course. It may present with dementia or focal lesions.

Encephalitis may be part of Cytomegalo Virus or Varicella zoster virus infection. Definite diagnosis, employing viral specific PCR for CSF samples, is essential. Different levels of *neuropathy, peripheral, multiple and/or autonomic*, is part of the HIV/AIDS complex. Peripheral neuropathy may be a side effect of different drug regimens.

Co-Infection of HIV and Hepatitis B Virus (HBV)

Co-infection of HIV and Hepatitis virus is common, since both share some routes of sexual and blood borne transmission. Patients coming from high prevalent areas (e.g., sub-Saharan Africa, south-east Asia), intravenous drug users (IDUs) and some haemophiliacs are high risk groups. With HIV co-infection, there is a high level of HBV Viraemia, rapid progress of cirrhosis and anti-retroviral hepato-toxicity. At the later stage of CD4 decline, chronic HBV infection may occur. Patients with higher CD4 count have a chance of HBV spontaneous recovery.

The aim of management is to suppress viral replication as cure is not achievable in most cases. The management of HBV and HIV co-infection requires multi-disciplinary team with special expertise. HIV patients on HAART are prone to hepato toxicity; therefore, liver function tests should be monitored closely. The treatment regimens include Pegylated Interferon, Emtricitabine, Lamivudine, Tenofovir, Adefovir and Entecavir. Pegylated Interferon could be used early, preferably prior to the need of HAART. The level of HBV – DNA and liver function dictate the start of treatment. Treatment should be part of HAART regimens (e.g., Lamivudine, Tenofovir, or Emtricitabine).

Patient at risk groups should be offered Hepatitis A and B vaccination at the earliest opportunity e.g., men having sex with men, intravenous drug users and those from high prevalence areas. HIV patients should be offered repeated tests for Hepatitis serology; between other STIs.

Co-Infection of HIV and Hepatitis C Virus (HCV)

HCV prevalence is higher in patients infected with HIV (affecting 1 in 10 patients). The rates are higher in IDUs and haemophiliacs, who are HIV positive. The clinical features are those of HCV infection. There doesn't appear to be a worsening of the HIV status, although the CD4 response to HAART is lower. The management of Hepatitis C and HIV co-infection require multi-disciplinary team with special skills. Treatment of HCV, if required, should be initiated prior to the need for HAART. HCV management follow the same lines for mono-infection (Pegylated, Alpha Interferon and Ribavirin). The response in delaying the progression of liver disease is better with genotype II and III but sustained viral response is achievable only in two-thirds of patients (one-third with genotype I). There is the option of liver transplantation, but would require a stable HIV status.

HIV and Pregnancy

Pre-conception counselling should aim to help the couple understand the relationship between HIV and pregnancy and to reach an informed choice. Artificial insemination is an option of the HIV-positive woman with an HIV-negative male partner. The sperm washing technique separates spermatozoa from seminal plasma and is used to inseminate the HIV-negative female partner of an HIV-positive male. The risk of transmission is estimated at 1:500 unprotected sexual acts. National antenatal screening for HIV helps to identify patients during early pregnancy. Index patient contact tracing is preferable, but the medical establishment has a professional responsibility for provider contact tracing, and patient's co-operation is therefore important. Management of HIV during pregnancy requires multidisciplinary teams with special expertise, including an obstetricians, HIV physician, paediatrician and a midwife. A maternity unit with specialised HIV expertise, where available, is ideal.

Mother to Child Transmission

Vertical HIV transmission varies from 1 in 5, in non breast feeding, to 1 in 3 in breast feeding. The chance of vertical transmission is higher in parallel with high maternal viral load. Vaginal delivery, chorioamnionitis, pre-term delivery and duration between rupture of membranes and delivery are risk factors for HIV transmission. The risk of vertical transmission has been reduced to 2% by anti-retroviral therapy to the mothers during pregnancy and labour; and to the newborn during the first 6 weeks of life. Caesarean delivery and avoidance of breast feeding contribute to the reduced transmission.

Clinical Practicalities

1. Both partners should be advised to take tests to exclude other STIs; including Syphilis, Hepatitis B and C, Gonorrhoea and Chlamydia.
2. There is a poor correlation between seminal and serum viral load level (ie a low level in serum may not correlate with that of the seminal fluid).
3. Couples who are both infected with HIV carry a risk of transmission of a drug resistant HIV strain, to either partners and the future child.
4. HIV sexual transmission must be emphasised, to avoid further transmission, following the diagnosis.
5. HIV monitoring and treatment follows general guidance. Repeat CD4 and Viral load tests identify the point at which therapy should start.
6. Opportunistic infections can readily develop during pregnancy and the threshold for therapy should start earlier.

HIV Therapy

The introduction of Highly Active Anti-Retroviral Therapy (HAART) has reduced HIV mortality and morbidity, improved prognosis and reduced opportunistic infections (OIs). Therapy initiation requires a balance between unnecessary early treatment and long-term drug side effects; and avoidance of late treatment when immunological damage may have taken place. The drug resistance profile should guide treatment. A frank, early discussion of pros and cons of therapy should be part of the post-test counselling. The patient should have the information and time to make an informed decision about therapy.

The point of starting therapy is a balance between rate of decline in CD4, rate of increase in viral load and patient's preference. The Acute Immunodeficiency associated with some primary HIV infections, can lead to opportunistic infections characteristic of late HIV and/or AIDS (e.g., PCP), and would require HAART. Symptomatic disease or a rapid progressive course will also require HAART. The speed at which immunodeficiency may develop in the older age group should be considered for earlier therapy. HAART is better delayed in cases where opportunistic or concurrent infections (PCP or TB) are requiring therapy, to avoid drug interactions and/or Immune-reconstitution effects. The drug therapy of these conditions should be initiated first. When the condition is under control, then HAART therapy is started. If HAART therapy is initiated at the same time, the improvement in immune functions and the Immune Reconstitution Syndrome may worsen the clinical condition (e.g., increased swelling and compression in a tuberculouss abscess).

The mechanism of action of anti-retroviral drugs depends on interrupting the viral replication process. Drugs aim to interrupt viral fusion with CD4 cells, integration of viral DNA with host cell DNA, reverse transcription of single strand RNA into double strand DNA; or protease processing of viral proteins.

The combination therapy should benefit from synergistic or additive activity; which should reduce the development of drug resistance. The clinician should avoid additive toxicity between combination drugs. There are three main sub-groups of drugs in clinical practice that intercept the HIV life cycle within the CD4 cells; eventually blocking different parts of the HIV life cycle and the production of virus copies. The integrase inhibitors block the virus integration into the CD4 cells DNA.

a. Fusion inhibitors interrupt the entry of the virus into the CD4 cell [T-20 blocks viral proteins from attaching to the cells' surface and CCR5 inhibitors block viral attachment to a core receptor].
b. Nucleoside and nucleotide reverse transcriptase inhibitors (NRTIs and NNRTIs) intercept the change of the HIV single strand of RNA into a double strand of DNA.

c.   The protease inhibitors (PI) intercept the assembly of the viral amino-acid chain into the right structure (leading into ineffective viral particles).

The standard choice for combination treatment is 2 NRTIs plus boosted PI, or 2 NRTIs plus a NNRTI. Most HIV treatment-naïve patients are started on Efavirenz or Nevirapine. Three drug therapy (triple therapy), and occasionally four drugs (quadruple therapy), have the benefit of intercepting viral replication at several points in the HIV multiplication cycle; whilst using sub-toxic dosages of drugs. The availability of several drugs within each group betters the choice to balance patients' convenience, drug side effect and tolerability

Clinical Practicalities

1.   Antiretroviral therapy does not cure HIV infection but increases the patient's life expectancy.
2.   The aim of treatment is to reduce HIV Viral Load as much, and for as long, as possible.
3.   Patients' compliance and adherence to therapy is of paramount importance for the control and long-term benefits of HIV therapy. The clinician should introduce information about therapy (verbal and written) to the patient at the earliest opportunity.
4.   The progressive reduction in bill burden and drug frequency is receiving welcoming approval from patients, due to increasing opinions.
5.   Patient's convenience and tolerance of side-effects plays a significant part in compliance with therapy.
6.   The deterioration of clinical condition and/or caused increase in Viral Load may require switching therapy or adding another HAART; the choice of which depends on the existing regimen, drug tolerance and cross-resistance.
7.   The teratogenic potential of most HAART is unknown. The HIV treatment for pregnant women aims at reducing disease progression, Viral Load and consequently transmission to foetus.
8.   HIV disease in children requires expertise of a multi-disciplinary team, preferably in a network of specialists.
9.   The use of antiretroviral drugs for PEP is an unlicensed indication.

Post-Exposure Prophylaxis (PEP)

Post-exposure Prophylaxis (PEP) entails the intake of anti-retroviral therapy, following a potential exposure to the HIV virus, to eliminate or reduce the opportunity of infection.

The clinical indications for PEP are: sexual exposure with a known partner (e.g., discordant sexual partnership), sexual transmission with unknown partner (e.g., sexual assault and rape), casual sexual intercourse in the high risk group (e.g., men having sex with men from a high risk area) or professional exposure (e.g., healthcare worker/needle-stick injury).

The chance of transmission, during professional exposure or sexual intercourse, increases with a breach in the integrity of the muco-cutaneous coverage, (e.g., wounds, abrasions, cuts, eczema), increased viral load in the index patient and/or the presence of other STIs (e.g., ulcerative genital disease).

Clinical Practicalities for PEP

1. The sero-prevalence of HIV in men having sex with men in high risk areas may reach 1 in 5.
2. The risk of transmission following needle-stick injury is estimated as 3 per 1000 injuries.
3. The risk statistics are relative. Some patients find comfort in taking the PEP to abate anxiety. The clinician must explain the pros and cons of transmission and drug side effects. The final decision is a patient privilege.
4. If the index case is known and willing to provide a blood sample for testing, a negative result would avoid the unnecessary intake of PEP. A designated health care professional (not the patient/health professional incurring the injury) should provide the counselling for the HIV testing, to avoid conflicts of interest or the index case feeling pressurised.
5. If there is a possibility of delay in obtaining the HIV result of the index case, the first dosage of PEP could be given to avoid delay in initiation of therapy.
6. The injured party may wish to have more time, to way up the pros and cons of treatment. The first dose of the PEP could be initiated at the earliest opportunity, until the patient reaches the final conclusion.

7. The window period between exposure and initiation of PEP is considered to be in the region of 2-3 days, but some patients may wish to start at a later time.
8. There have been instances where PEP has failed to prevent HIV infection following occupational exposure, which should be explained to the patient.
9. Neonates given 6 weeks' course of Zidovudine, initiated within 48 hours of delivery, had a protective effect against transmission (from HIV positive mothers who did not receive anti-retroviral therapy before delivery).
10. Viral resistance plays a part in the efficacy of the Prophylaxis (e.g., if the virus transmitted is resistant to one or more of the PEP drugs). If the pattern of viral resistance in the index case is known, the PEP regimen should be devised accordingly.
11. Adherence and compliance with PEP is poor.
12. The use of antiretroviral drugs for PEP is an unlicensed indication.

Drug Regimens Recommended for PEP

Zidovudine (AZT) has been studied with evidence showing reduction in risk of HIV transmission following exposure; therefore, should be considered in the regimen (unless there is evidence of AZT viral resistance).

The regimen options include: Zidovudine (300 mg) and Lamivudine (150 mg), plus Nelfinavir (1.25 g) twice daily. Alternatives for Zidovudine are Stavudine (30-40 mg twice daily, according to patient's weight), Tenofovir (300 mg, once daily). Either drug is used in addition to Lamivudine and Nelfinavir.

Practical Considerations for PEP

1. Three drugs are more effective than one.
2. The local patterns of drug resistance should influence therapeutic options for PEP.
3. Abacavir is better avoided as first-line therapy due to its high hypersensitivity reactions.
4. Nevirapine has high rates of hepatotoxicity and a potential for fulminate hepatic failure and is better avoided as first choice.

5. Efavirenz is better avoided due to its psychotropic effects and drug reactions (e.g., rash); both cause patients anxiety and are unjustifiable for a short course of treatment.

6. Emergency services should co-operate in setting guidelines of concerted effort to deal with PEP (Accident and Emergency, Microbiology, Infectious Diseases and HIV Medicine Departments).

7. The patient should be made aware of the lack of data on the efficacy of PEP.

8. Lack of compliance could be reduced by adequate counselling prior to the initiation of PEP and follow-up to deal with side effects and/or anxieties, possibly on a weekly basis.

9. An Antibody test should be ordered 3 and 6 months following exposure; to ascertain the patient status and efficacy of PEP.

10. Occupational exposure should be followed by a blood sample, obtained early to ascertain the patient's status at that point of time. Failed PEP and the acquisition of HIV constitutes industrial injury, with its legal and insurance ramifications.

HIV Drug Therapy

A) Non-Nucleoside Reverse Transcriptase Inhibitors (NNRTIs)

DRUG	DOSAGE	SIDE EFFECTS / TOXICITY	ADVANTAGES
Efavirenz (EFZ)	600 mg once daily	Drug teratogenicity (contra-indicated in pregnancy), Hepatitis and CNS effects	1. Patients' convenience for once daily dosage and low pill burden. 2.Less lipodystrophy and lipid problems.
Nevirapine (NVP)	400mg once or 200 mg twice daily	Hepatitis, Stevens-Johnson Syndrome and skin rash	DISADVANTAGES: 1. Inherent resistance against HIV-2. 2. Single mutations lead to resistance within the group.
Delavirdine (DLV)	400 mg three times daily	Skin reactions and Diarrhoea.	

B) Nucleoside Reverse Transcriptase Inhibitors (NRTIs)

DRUG	DOSAGE	SIDE EFFECTS / TOXICITY	ADVANTAGES
Abacavir (ABC)	300mg twice daily	Life-threatening hypersensitivity reactions, pyrexia, lethargy and gastrointestinal symptoms	
Didanosine (DDI)	300-400 mg once daily depending on weight	Pancreatitis, Lactic Acidosis pose a serious risk.Peripheral Neuropathy, Hepatic Steatosis, nausea and diarrhoea	
Emtricitabine (FTC)	200 mg once daily	Lactic Acidosis, Hepatic Steatosis	
Lamivudine (3TC)	300 mg once daily or 150 mg twice daily	Lactic Acidosis, Hepatic Steatosis	
Stavudine (D4T)	30 mg – 40 mg twice daily depending on weight	Lipodystrophy, Peripheral Neuropathy, pancreatitis, lactic Acidosis, Hepatic Steatosis	
Alcitapine (EDC)	0.75 mg three times daily	Peripheral Neuropathy,	
Zidovudine (AZT)	250–300mg twice daily	Pancreatisis, Stomatitis, Lactic Acidosis, Hepatic Steatosis Bone Marrow suppression, Myopathy, Lactic Acidosis, Hepatic Steatosis	

C) Nucleotide Reverse Transcriptase Inhibitor (NRTI)

DRUG	DOSAGE	SIDE EFFECTS / TOXICITY	ADVANTAGES
Tenofovir	300 mg once daily	Renal insufficiency, asthenia, gastrointestinal symptoms and headache	

D) Protease Inhibitors (PIs)

DRUG	DOSAGE	SIDE EFFECTS / TOXICITY	ADVANTAGES
Amprenavir (APV)	600 mg twice daily	Lipodystrophy,gastrointestinal disturbances, skin rash, oral paraesthesia	1) Lower class and genetic resistance. 2) Lower skin & hepatic reactions.
Atazanavir (ATZ)	300 mg daily	Hyperbilirubinaemia, cardiac conduction effect	DISADVANTAGES:
Fosamprenavir (FPV)	700 mg twice daily	Lipodystrophy,gastrointestinal disturbances, skin rash	1)High drug inter-actions 2) Require food & drink restrictions with high bill burden.
Indinavir (IDV)	800 mg twice daily	Lipodystrophy, Hyperbilirubinaemia, gastrointestinal disturbances, Nephrolithiasis	3) Lipodystrophy & hyperlipidaemia.
Lopinavir (LPV) with Ritonavir (RTV)	LPV 200 mg, RTV 50 mg 2 tab.twice daily	Lipodystrophy,gastrointestinal disturbances, Asthenia, raised transaminases.	
Saquinavir	1 g twice daily	Lipodystrophy, gastrointestinal disturbances, raised transaminases	
Ritonavir	Initially 300 mg twice daily, increased in steps of 100 mg every 12 hours to 600 mg twice daily	Lipodystrophy, Pancreatisis, Hepatitis, gastrointestinal disturbances, paraesthesia, raised transaminases	
Nelfinavir (NFV)	1.25 g twice daily	Lipodystrophy, diarrhoea, increased transaminases	
Ritonavir (RTV) To boost other PIs	100 mg twice daily to boost other PI or 100 mg daily with AZT		

E) Fusion Inhibitor (FI)

DRUG	DOSAGE	SIDE EFFECTS / TOXICITY	ADVANTAGES
Enfuvrtide (ENF)	90 mg twice daily Subcutaneous injections	Hypersensetivity	Used in other drug treatment failure

About the Author

A.R. Markos FRCOG FRCP
Consultant in Genitourinary Medicine& Sexual Health
Stafford, UK.

The Sexually Transmitted Infections book provides an overall practical account for the benefit of generalists and Primary Care physicians, who would encounter the patients' problems first; and those intending to specialise. The emphasis on clinical issues is drawing from the author's 30 years of progressive clinical experience in Primary Care, Urology, Obstetrics and Gynaecology and Venereology. Patients who wish to acquire unbiased in depth knowledge about sexually transmitted infections, will find answers to their questions. Many of these questions were asked times and times again by patients who shared similar concerns and anxieties.

The book covers a wide range of clinical practices and facilities and addresses areas of low resource settings, which will make the account relevant to developing primary health units.

Index

C

D

N

T

U